JEN
GROTHE

75 WAYS TO LOVE YOUR OATMEAL
AND OTHER TREATS, TIPS & TRICKS

Published by Sound Concepts
782 South Auto Mall Drive, Suite A
American Fork, UT 84003
Visit us at: Jen-Fit-Books.com

Design by: Sound Concepts
Recipe photos by: Camille Funk

ISBN: 978-1-936631-02-5

Jenny's Contact Information:

Email: jen.fit.training@gmail.com

Blog: Jen-Fit's Fitness and Recipe Blog
http://jen-fit-training.blogspot.com/

Facebook group: Recipes for Gals in Figure &
Bodybuilding
http://www.facebook.com/RecipesforGals

Website: Jen-Fit, Inc.
www.jen-fit.com

Important: The information in this book reflects the author's experiences and opinions and is not intended to replace medical advice.

Before beginning this or any nutritional or exercise regimen, consult your physician to be sure it is appropriate for you. Ask for a physical stress test.

TABLE OF CONTENTS

Dedication 5

Acknowledgement 7

Testimonials From Facebook Fans........................ 9

My Story 19

Make One Small Change 39

The Importance of Breakfast............................51

Why Oatmeal?...55

What's in my Fridge and in my Pantry.................59

My Favorite Products & Where to Find Them 61

My Life Then & My Life Now 65

The Health Benefits of Eating Clean 69

Oatmeal Recipes..73

A Q&A with Jenny Grothe................................177

Recommended Reading and Sites.......................187

About the Author...189

Recipe Index..191

DEDICATION:

If *you* would have told me three years ago I was starting a new journey,
I never would have known to what extent.

If *you* would have told me that only three years later I would have dropped 60
pounds and been healthier than I was as a teenager,
I would have thought you were a dreamer.

If *you* would have told me back then that one day I'd be on stage
in front of thousands of people in next to barely nothing,
I would have laughed at you.

If *you* would have told me that I, Jenny Grothe,
would one day bring home a trophy (let alone 5) because of my physique,
I would have thought it was a sick joke.

If *you* would have told me back in the day when I skipped school
in order to not have to run the mile,
that one day I'd qualify and be running the Boston Marathon,
I would have doubted you.

...and if *you* would have told me a year ago I'd be publishing my first cookbook,
I wouldn't have believed you.

Yet here *I am.*

So this book is dedicated to the *you* in all of us,
to my kids, Dakota and Zane, and to all the non-believers out there.

This is for all the *I can not* and the *I will never* excuses.
That turned into *I can* and *I will* commitments.

ACKNOWLEDGEMENTS:

I'd like to make special mention of a few key people who've had a positive impact on me during my weight-loss journey. Each one of them has helped me and continues to help me in some way. Their encouragement, love, and support helps make me stronger.

First and foremost I want to thank my wonderful, loving, and supportive husband. He has never doubted me. He loved me before, and he loves me now.

I'd also like to thank my loving family and supportive friends.

In the industry, I'd like to thank LuAnn, Sandy, Mike, Scott, and Landon. You know who you are. I'll always be a work in progress but because of your knowledge and direction, you're helping me get there. Thank you.

TESTIMONIALS FROM FACEBOOK FANS

Sarah Dunstan (VA) - Jen has taken the art of oatmeal preparation to a whole new level! Now a bland, but nutritious staple food has taken on a whole new life and flavor of its own thanks to Jen's creativity. There is something for everyone and every age here. These recipes will delight year round. Jen has found a way to get everyone to Eat their Oatmeal! And love it!

Pascale Digioia (FL) - I love Jen's daily oatmeal and breakfast recipes! Every day when I log onto Facebook, she always has an amazing, healthy, low-fat recipe, perfect for a diet where you are preparing for fitness or bodybuilding. I have tried several already and my favorite is by far the oatmeal chocolate chip protein muffins––they are to die for! I bake my muffins early so I have them on hand anytime I have a craving. I'm a chocoholic on a diet, so I just want to say, "Thank you Jen for your amazing recipes! You rock, girl!"

Rebecka Tobler (Switzerland) - I look forward to some new recipe ideas from Jen daily. You don't have to be a bodybuilder to enjoy these low-fat, high-protein dishes! Lots of times I see combinations of ingredients I have never seen before and I am amazed at the amazing flavors that can be experienced!

Jen is doing us ladies (and gents) a huge favor with her fun recipes! I have experienced new joy in cooking through Jen's recipes! All I can say is bravo for all the effort she puts into getting the recipes out to us and a big thank you for bringing us such tasty and healthy alternatives!

Brenda Argraves - I enjoy reading your posts on a daily basis. They encourage me to continue to fight to be the best I can be. It is nice to see the honest, day-to-day goings-on in your life. It makes me feel like you are not some celebrity fitness guru, but someone I can relate to! I enjoy your recipes and have tried some of them with success. I enjoyed the baked strawberry cream cheese oatmeal a lot. Thanks for the encouragement!

Lisa Godfrey (MO) - I found Jen's site on Facebook just by accident six or eight months ago. I immediately fell in love with it because she truly cares about fitness and putting out the best information and recipes that she can find for the followers. I have tried so many of her recipes that she now has her own section in my cookbook! They are all healthy (and if not, she makes sure to warn you in advance!) and very good taste-wise. I have been trying to eat more healthy and found that many of the recipes are tasteless, but not Jen's!

I have found inspiration for my own weight loss journey by reading her struggles, setbacks and her eventual triumph with her weight. I love reading her posts about her family and how she gets them involved in fitness and health. She seems to be a genuinely good-hearted person and I admire her courage to put herself out there for all of us!

Cristina Hagerty - I want to tell you how much you inspire me. You make me believe. I want to thank God for bringing you into my life even though I have never met you in person. I already started my journey, and I understand I have a long way to go, but I will get there, I know it! Keep up the wonderful work, and perhaps I will meet you one day, and thank you in person!

Marlo Maxwell - I feel like I owe you so much for all you have done for me in the past six months or so. I have learned so much about how I want to be, and how I don't have to live my life in the extreme, like I have pretty much all my life. I was a collegiate athlete and I trained for fitness comps when I was 19. When I graduated I thought, "I can finally do nothing!" I let the athlete inside of me die when I got married and quickly had kids, thinking that I was selfish to want more than the many blessings I have. It took some devastating family tragedies, back-to-back, to make me see that life is so short, and that sitting around being a martyr for fear of being myself was wasteful and not at all what God would want from me. I am so thankful that you have shown me how being a great mom goes hand in hand with taking care of yourself, and keeping your own goals on the priority list. You rock my socks off.

Marianna Clark - Thanks Jen! You put an enormous amount of time and work into a FB page and blog for thousands of people you don't even know. You are really paying it forward the way God would want us to.

After my first child I worked out, but after I had my second child, I had extra weight I couldn't lose. I was putting everyone else ahead of me, and not taking the time to really take care of myself. I packed on pounds after Alexis was born by eating fast food for lunch every day because I didn't have time to pack my lunch. I quit weighing myself at 180, but my weight gain didn't stop there, and I haven't had my picture taken voluntarily since my daughter was born in March of 2008. I stumbled across your page by accident, and when I read your story, it really hit home with me. I made a decision then and there that I was going to make the time and effort to start taking care of me, as well as my family. I am down to 160, with a lot more to go, but it is because of your story. You put yourself out there, and let people know it can be done. Whenever I feel like I can't do it, or it can't be done, I think of you. I know that if you did it, with all of the other commitments you have in your life, that I can definitely do it. You are a woman who has been in my shoes, and knows what I am going through, and you brought yourself through it to the amazing place you are today. You have given me my life back, and for that I am eternally grateful to you.

Jan Petersen - Thank you so much Jen. You are always helping me make better choices. If you only knew how much you truly help so many. I love seeing what you are making, or doing first thing in morning. I am working to lose a lot of weight. In fact your story sounds much like mine. I'm 36 and need to lose 40 pounds. I gained it after a miscarriage. I just gave up. I know it is possible to do this because I see you.

Jennifer Bower (CO) - Jenny has been a wonderful inspiration to me. There are foods out there that I would have never heard of and they are now staples in my pantry and kitchen. I was already eating clean prior to stumbling upon her Facebook page. Finding her was like opening another door into my clean eating lifestyle. The oatmeal bars and shakes never cease to make my muscles and body crave them. Just when I thought I was at my best fitness/lifestyle-wise, I discovered Jen's site and was reawakened with new ideas, tools, inspiration and motivation to strive to be even better. I find myself at my gym talking about Jen like she is truly my gal-friend. When I'm shopping and buying certain products I suggest to the cashier or anyone near me how they can use that in a way you would have never thought--thanks to Jen. When I first wake up early in the morning I am always excited and eager to wonder, "What is Jen going to post this morning?" Thank you Jen for all that you do for all of us "fit-gals"!

Tracie Elias (IL) - I started a new clean eating plan for my life a couple months ago. I am constantly searching for support and new, simple clean eating recipes for my family on the Internet. Somehow I came across Jen's site through Facebook. It was the best find ever! I just told my hubby today that when I am spending too much time on Facebook, I am not even looking at friend's photos or reading their posts; I am reading on Jen's site for all her yummy and super-simple recipes! Once I started reading through them and trying some, I found myself sincerely hoping that she would have an actual cookbook! I have been eating oatmeal every day now for the first time in my life and love to keep making new flavors to keep it fun. I will be the first in line to purchase Jen's oatmeal cookbook and any more recipe books to come.

Cynthia Bazin (NV) - Recently I have had the opportunity to connect with Jenny Grothe. I wish I knew her years ago! As a fitness enthusiast, I am always looking for great healthy recipes to make as I train, and she has the absolute best recipes! Jenny is so creative––the ingredient combination in her recipes is amazing, and the finished product is always so delicious! One of my favorite recipes is her Baked Oatmeal. Absolutely awesome!

Calee Creer - I check Jen's recipe site every day and every time I'm always pleased with what I find! The baked oatmeal is easy and so good. I've bookmarked the recipes and can't wait for a cookbook! Jen is an awesome athlete and such an inspiration. I look forward to the great things she has in store!

Debra Curry (MD) - I just wanted to say how much I love all of your recipes. As a Certified Personal Trainer, I love sharing them with my clients as healthier options for meals and snacks. Your oatmeal recipes are so delicious and keep my morning meals from getting too boring. Your spirit and uplifting comments keep all of us positive and ready to tackle the day. Thanks for all of your recipes and a blog that helps to educate along with having some fun!

50 -Year-Old "Nana" - Thank you for all the motivation and yummy recipes! You have helped this 50-year-old nana get herself going again. Please keep posting; I'm so glad I found you.

Carmen Robinson - Trying to eat a clean bodybuilder's diet is a very difficult task because there are only so many things we can regularly eat and apparently only so many different ways to cook them. That's where Jen comes in. She is extremely creative in coming up with ways to cook healthy meals in delicious ways. She is willing to experiment and then share her creations and even comes up with the macros so we know exactly what we are getting. Every one of her recipes is clearly written so it is easy to follow and the results have never disappointed me—always a hit! And her recipes are so good that the rest of the family happily eats them too. I am very grateful to have her in my life as I pursue my fitness goals.

Jillian Schofield - I'm a physical therapist and baked oatmeal has become one of my staples! I have always enjoyed oats, but after trying it baked, I was hooked! I rave about it and share the recipes with all of my patients! I have even had several patients that say they hate oatmeal, and then try it this way, and now like it! I look forward to baked oatmeal every week! You and your recipes have become a huge part of my lifestyle change and I'm so grateful I found you.

Jen Cooder - You are an inspiration. I love your recipes. I look them up to get new healthy ideas to cook with. I love your oatmeal recipes––you got me hooked on the stuff and now I love it.

Becky Brown - I am a dancer. I have been using and loving your daily recipes. I actually wake up early like you, so I love the fact that at 4 a.m. you've posted my newest favorite recipes. I use your oatmeal recipes every day, mainly because I love oatmeal, but I also love the variations. Thank you for the healthy, amazing, yummy, and informative site.

Wendy Moore - Jen's oatmeal recipes can be enjoyed for breakfast, lunch, dinner or an evening snack. Who would have ever thought that something so delicious and simple to make could be so healthy for you? My husband, who swore he would never eat oatmeal, has been truly won over by the Baked Berry Oatmeal. Thank you for inspiring all of us each day to eat healthy.

Linda Bettencourt - I appreciate all of your recipes, the clean-eating advice, and most of all, your positive attitude. You've given me so many great healthy cooking ideas. I can honestly say that the reason I check my Facebook every day is to read your posts. I competed this July and my diet was so much easier, thanks to your great recipes! You are such an inspiration to fitness, and a beautiful person inside and out!

Valerie Sayer (Canada) - Oatmeal has always been a staple in my house but now with your baked oatmeal recipes our love for it has been taken to a whole new level! The blueberry cheesecake recipe is the favorite in our household—and in fact, when I make it for friends, they immediately ask for the recipe too! Thank you Jen for giving my family tasty recipes—they truly are a gift of healthy living!

Briana Brumfield (OK) Ever since coming across your page a few months ago, I have found myself over-the-top obsessed with baking! I can't even walk into my house without turning the oven on right away because I know I'm going to be cooking something! After eating extremely clean and with little variety for over two years, your recipes have opened my eyes to new, delicious entrees, oatmeals, and shakes that meet my strict macro levels and coincide with my lifestyle and the way I like to eat. Being only 19, I'm one in a dozen who would rather spend my free time baking the newest protein bar recipe rather than being out at the bars or stuffing their faces with pizza and nachos. I have your site bookmarked on my phone and pull it up every day and I can't get enough! Your page has sparked my overly indulgent obsession with baking. Thanks for everything! You're awesome and such an inspiration to women everywhere!

Tracy Gonsalves (UT) - Your oatmeal recipes have helped me feed my husband a hearty nutrient-packed breakfast in the morning with sustainable carbs and protein and without excessive calories. He is a recuperating paraplegic and needs to put muscle back on—but his legs won't support carrying around the extra weight that just plain old calorie-dense food will put on. I am always looking for a way to find thought-out calories, which is where your recipes have been perfect. (Plus they're great for my figure too!!)

Jennifer Hugunin - I could not live without your recipes! They are all quick, easy, delicious, and super healthy. Whenever I need a recipe idea, your page is my first stop. What I especially love is that people have tried the recipes and added input to make it better, and that you have the nutritional info listed. Your recipes helped me reach my goal of winning my first figure competition. Your recipe ideas made my bland, boring figure diet delicious and enjoyable. Thanks. I couldn't have done it without you!

Ellen Holmes, NPC Figure Competitor - I see you on FB all the time! I've made so many of your recipes! Your oatmeal recipes are my faves, especially those soft protein bars. I make a batch for my trainer every Friday to keep him in line.

I have to say, those oatmeal recipes have been the highlight of my meal plans. How can something that tastes like dessert be so good for you? I've always liked oatmeal, even as a kid, but day after day, even oatmeal gets boring. I was eating oatmeal every morning before training to give me the carbs I needed to get through the training; it really works! Then I saw your recipe on FB for the oatmeal with the egg whites, protein powder and SF maple syrup, and I was hooked! Tastes like dessert, but packs a good punch in the gym!

For me, oatmeal is one of the mainstays of my diet—I bring the protein bars with me to shows, even, to keep me looking full! YUM!

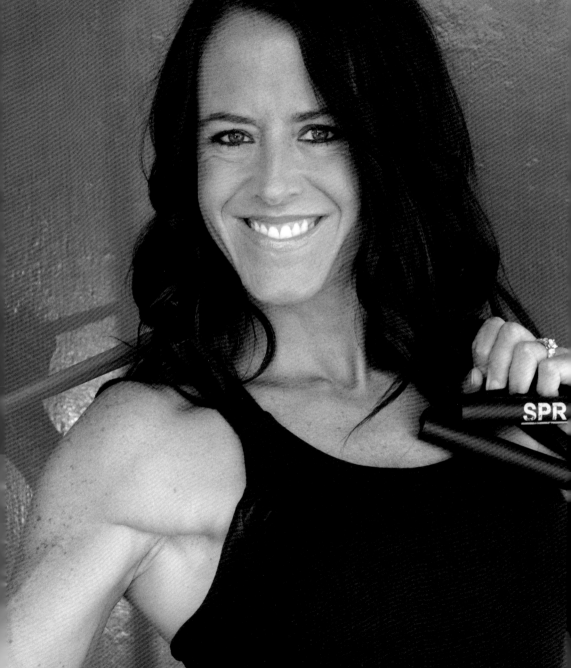

You say I can't? **I say I can.**

You think it won't happen? **I know it will.**

You say never? **I say wait and see.**

You think I'm wasting my time? **I'll show you I'm not.**

You question why? **I answer why not try?**

– Jenny Grothe

MY STORY

My name is **Jenny Grothe.**

Some of you are familiar with my story. I'm guessing the majority of you are not.

Three years ago I was 170 pounds and a size 14. That was September 2007—really not that long ago. Now thinking back I can't believe how much has changed in such a short period of time. I am a completely different person now. I was always the same on the inside, but I'm now the happier, more confident, driven, courageous, energetic me that I was when I was younger.

I was slim growing up. Not overly slim, but I didn't have any weight issues. I'll tell you that. I was active in school. I participated in sports. I was on the drill team, and I felt confident strutting my stuff across the stage in a cherry red evening gown and three-inch heels for Jazz choir. I was confident.
I never worked out.

I didn't watch what I ate.

Sports to me were sports and nothing more. I never consciously worked out. I didn't think about adding muscle, cardio, or watching what I ate. I didn't have to.

Of course being a girl, I still gossiped with my friends in the hall about other girls, what they wore, how they looked, and evaluated every single thing. The same went for me. I'd critique myself. I knew others were doing the same thing. They were critiquing me. Sadly, that's just what girls do. So, like every other girl, I always felt like I should be on a diet. Back then being on a diet meant eating less candy, skipping a meal, or using it as an excuse not to eat a dinner. It wasn't that I needed to diet. I was just being a typical girl.

As a senior I remember going to the doctor for a physical. I don't remember much about my visits to the doctor as a youth, but I do remember that one in particular. My doctor mentioned I had "great birthing hips." "Uh, thanks. What's that supposed to mean? Great birthing hips? You mean my hips are wide? What?" That was the first time someone else ––and in this case, someone of a respectable authority, hinted to me that I had a weight problem. Looking back and now knowing what I know, I didn't have a weight problem at that time, but his statement still left me feeling crushed and insecure.

I was 118 pounds, and I had "great birthing hips." Time passed.

Another incident happened when I was in college. My best friend Cami and I took a modeling class. I never felt like a model, but we both thought it would be a fun after-school activity, and why not pretend?

The class really was fun. We got to dress up, learn proper etiquette, learn how to do our hair and makeup (granted it was the 80s, so in order to do our hair, we simply had to tease it higher), and practice our walks for the runway.

Then we had our one-on-one meetings with our teacher.

"Jenny, your thighs touch. We can't be having that." What? My thighs touch? All of the sudden I was aware that my thighs actually rubbed when I walked. I'd never even noticed that before. I evaluated the star pupil of the class—the teacher's pet. Her thighs didn't touch. But mine did. Every. Single. Step.

I was 121 pounds, but my thighs touched.

That was just the beginning. I share this because as women we are surrounded by unfair expectations. Basically we are told our bodies are not good enough when in reality they are. Based on society, we are supposed to be taller, thinner, and lighter, and look a certain way. It starts early. The expectations to be skinnier are always there.

My 20s were pretty uneventful body-image-wise.

Greg and I marred in 1991. We moved to Utah. We earned five dollars an hour at our jobs. We both worked at the same company––I worked early mornings; he worked afternoons and evenings. We rarely saw each other. When we weren't working we went to school. We lived in an apartment across the street from Wal-Mart. We ate what we could afford, and that wasn't much. We stocked up on frozen burritos, shoestring French fries, store brand chicken potpies, and soda. Our dinners out included frequent visits to Taco Bell where we purchased whatever we could buy from their 59-cent menu.

As newlyweds we had no one hanging over our shoulders telling us what we could and could not do. I'd never lived outside my mom and dad's house until I was married. Without any prior college experience to prep me, I went straight from my parents to married life, which meant I had a newfound freedom that made me think I could now do things I couldn't do before. A lot of that freedom came in the form of food. We'd fill up our big jugs before work with fully loaded

"Whether you think you can or you think you can't, you're right."

– Henry Ford

caffeinated sugary drinks. We'd chug them all day long. On date night, we loved going to the drive-in double features. We'd pack our pillows and sleeping bags in the back of the pickup truck, and then stock up on all the goodies––bags of chips, cheese dip, salsa, a box of raspberry filled donuts, boxed candies, and our big 64 oz. containers of soda. It was ridiculous. Yet at the time we were young, our bodies were still burning through calories like crazy, and we had freedom. It was okay. We were only accountable to each other, and we were having a great time. As long as we weren't getting fat, who cared? We didn't even think twice about our diets. Ever.

It didn't catch up to us for a long time.

Then, one spring, my mom sent me the most beautiful Easter dress. It was gorgeous. It was completely modest, had an apricot colored chiffon rose in the front and it was the most beautiful dress I owned at the time. I certainly wasn't in the position to be buying new clothes for myself. We didn't have the money. I was so excited to receive this new addition from my mom.

But I couldn't zip it up. The dress was a junior size. Apparently, I wasn't.

Our 20s came and went quickly. Though I never saw a huge change on the scale, we had changed. Our habits had changed. Our lifestyles had changed. We spent our 20s building bad habits. We ate all the time or not at all. We "pigged out" by hitting cheap breakfast buffets. We didn't exercise. We didn't read labels. We didn't think about healthy options. We ate out of convenience and limited our menu options to food choices we could afford.

Then came our 30s. I remember so many people telling me, "it will catch up to you in your 30s." Yeah, right. Old wives' tale. What was so magical about my 30s?

By the time I entered my 30s my metabolism had slowed. After years and years of consuming unhealthy foods with very limited physical activity, my body didn't respond the way it had when I was younger. By this time Greg and I very rarely did anything active; we didn't take walks, we didn't go for jogs, and we didn't hike. We had never done any of those things. Neither one of us competed in city or church sports. We just continued with our same poor habits and our inactive lifestyles, watching our bodies slowly deteriorate, not really knowing what to do, but also not really wanting to change anything.

I weighed around 150 pounds.

It was about this time that I first looked at dieting seriously. There were so many options out there. Too many. Atkins. The Zone Diet. Weight Watchers. Jenny Craig. Low-carb this and high-protein that.

Greg and I decided to try the Atkins Diet. Since we were used to eating greasy fatty foods, the idea

> "Learn how to be happy with what you have while you pursue all that you want."

of being able to eat loads of eggs, cheese, burgers, and bacon really appealed to us––it kind of felt like we were able to have our cake and eat it too. Really? Lose weight by eating all fattening foods? Okay, sign me up! I omitted the carbs and focused on what was allowed. I saw immediate results and at first it felt too good to be true. It was. A few weeks into it I felt sick to my stomach. I felt sluggish, uncomfortable, and heavy. Not to mention the fact that I was tired of having to pee on a stick to see if I was in ketosis or not. That diet did not work for me. I gave up.

So then I attended Weight Watchers. Some family members had gone through that process, and had achieved great results. They could calculate what to eat and how much to eat and would even allow themselves little cheats here and there as long as they stayed within their points. I wanted to be able to do that. It seemed to be working, so why not? I went to my first meeting. I hate meetings.

Ever since Greg and I were first married, I'd worked. In school I was very driven, and that didn't change with my job. I quickly excelled at my job, found my niche, and climbed the corporate latter. I did well and made a lot of money–– especially for a woman. I worked in a white-collar office with extremely driven 20-something men. I was the outcast, so I had to work that much harder. I did. And I was rewarded. It meant the world to me at the time, but with the success came stress. With the stress came emotional eating and even less physical activity because I was tied to early and late hours at my office job. And with that job came hours and hours of meetings. I hate meetings.

When I found out Weight Watchers wanted to have weekly accountability meetings, I was completely turned off. You want me to do what? No thanks. I will say that Weight Watchers helped me realize how damaging soda can be. In the two weeks I was with Weight Watchers, I dropped 8 pounds cutting out soda. I believe a lot of that was water weight, but still. The soda had to go.

By this time I was around 160 pounds.

Then Body for Life came along. I bought the book. I looked through pages and pages of before and after pictures. Success stories. People who were bigger than me and had lost so much weight. The people had changed completely. You couldn't even recognize them. They looked fitter, younger, happier, and healthier. A lot of them had won some serious cash along the way. That could be me. That would be me. I dug out an old swimsuit, and I made Greg take pictures of me. I wanted to be a transformation success story. I wanted to lose a ton of weight, look fitter, younger, happier, and healthier. I wanted to win $10,000. I wanted to be on the inside of the book.

For the first time I learned about the importance of healthy dieting AND exercising. I'd never really paired them together before. I had an actual plan to follow. It was all about balance —moderate carbs, moderate proteins, and lower fat. I learned about eating five to six meals a day. That was new to me. I learned about healthy snacking options. I

"What we think,

we become."

learned about free days, which for me translated to eat-everything-you-can-fit-in-your-mouth days. This was the first time I'd found a diet that seemed doable and made sense. I didn't feel like I was too deprived. I felt energized, and since Greg and I did it together, we had each other for accountability. I wanted to lose weight, and Body for Life helped me do that. I dropped from 160 to 130. I felt incredible. It worked. I was lighter than I'd been in years. I felt prettier than I'd felt in years.

During this time we tried to get pregnant—to no avail. After several tests, we learned I couldn't have babies. My tubes were completely closed. We underwent surgery to open them back up. But it didn't work. We went through in vitro twice. That didn't work. My body rejected everything. It was a very taxing time for us emotionally. In my opinion, nothing makes you feel less of a woman than learning you can't have children naturally. That is something we are expected to do when we grow up. I wanted to be a mom so badly, and it never even struck me that I might not be able to have children of my own. After a few years of investigative surgery and fertility procedures, we turned to adoption. It was at that time we brought our baby Dakota into our home. We would not trade him for the world, but the years leading up to his adoption were extremely difficult in every way imaginable. My self-esteem went from okay to barely existent. I couldn't help but feel like I was a failure. Once again, I turned to emotional eating.

By the time we were finally able to bring Dakota into our home, I'd already quit my office job. I was now working from home for a publishing company. I loved it, and I loved being able to stay at home with my baby. My world revolved around him. I spent every waking hour caring for him, loving him, nurturing him, and giving him all that a mom could give. I didn't want to take this long-awaited

> "Persistence is the twin sister of excellence. One is a matter of quality; the other, a matter of time."

blessing for granted. The more time I focused on Dakota, the less time I took care of me.

My 30s were up and down. From time to time I tried to get back on the Body for Life bandwagon, but it would only be for brief periods of time. I'd be drained, and I'd turn to a bowl of ice cream. When we'd want to go out, we went to our favorite Mexican restaurant. Instead of working out, I'd take Dakota to the park. Instead of making healthy dinners, I'd make what Dakota would eat or what was fast. I'd eat when I could fit it in or not at all. The other extreme was I'd eat as much as I possibly could all at once out of stress. My 30s were an absolute joke health-wise. By my mid-30s I was back to where I was pre Body For Life––only this time worse.

By the summer of 2007 I was wearing a size 14 and weighed 170 pounds.

This is the part of my story that many of you have heard.

I was physically at my worst. By most people's standards, I was borderline fat. I hate to use that word, but I was. At the time I never really felt that way. I still tried to wear cute clothes. I took the time to put on my makeup just right, highlight my hair, and style it just the way I wanted. I knew I needed to lose weight. I wasn't oblivious to the scale, but I didn't realize just how much.

Then a series of events started to unfold, and they crept under my skin.

In our mid-30s we moved into a new neighborhood. We were within a couple of miles of where Greg went to school. We were back on his stomping grounds. We've always been active members of our church, but this neighborhood took "active" to an entirely new level. We moved in to our new home in the winter and were able to successfully hide away from our neighbors for a while. Then spring came around and that completely changed. We were wooed into doing things with our neighbors several times a week. Now that may seem like a lot, but it's exactly what we needed at the time. Both of us love to be around people, but it was just as easy for us to hide ourselves away. The longer we hid, the more anti-social we became. In reality, we needed others to help pull us out of our seclusion.

We became quick friends with a few families in our neighborhood. They were friendly, loving, charitable, service-oriented, and extremely outgoing. We learned quickly that they would do anything for us, and that their friendships were genuine. But all of the wives in our new circle were tiny. One was a size 0 (yes, that number does exist), one was a size 2, another a size 4, and the other a size 6. Then there was me. Jenny. Size 14. My size was more than the sum of all theirs. Why did they want to be friends with me?

They did though. Just like my wonderful husband, they loved me unconditionally.

Being a part of this active group meant I was now attempting to do things I hadn't done for years. They enjoyed camping, hiking, swimming, and playing with the kids outdoors. They helped me remember how fun it was to be youthful again.

During one our get-togethers we were playing tag in the backyard. We laid out several blankets on the grass. Everyone had to choose a blanket to stand on. One person was the shark. That person's job was to catch one of us as we scurried from one blanket to another. The goal was not to be caught. It was a fun game, and I remember my heart skipped a beat because being chased had always scared me as a kid. But it wasn't that that really made my heart stop. One of the husbands, a good friend of ours, mentioned under his breath, but just loud enough for me to overhear, "Are you sure Jenny will be able to do this?" It took me back to the day when I was told I had great birthing hips and back to the time when I was told my thighs touched. Up to that point I'd felt like my weight problem was just me. It was at that moment I realized other people noticed how big I was too.

"Never underestimate the power of dreams and the influence of the human spirit."

Shortly after that, the moms in this group decided it would be fun to take the kiddos to St. George for a quick getaway. One of our adventures would be hiking through the Small Narrows—a narrow crevice between two sides of the mountain. I was a little hesitant but excited at the same time. The kids practically ran through it––no problems whatsoever. The moms had to inch through sideways. I let them all go ahead of me, preferring to go last. I started through the narrow path at first with no problem. There were a couple of patches where it was pretty tight, but I was able to suck in and push through––fully knowing I was probably tearing up my clothes, but not wanting to be left behind. Then came an obstacle. I had to step up while on my side in a very narrow section of the path. I couldn't do it. I was stuck. I stayed there literally for minutes, sweat beading up on my face. I was embarrassed, scared, and was afraid they'd have to get help. This is not an exaggeration! At this point the other moms were still moving along through the narrows––they had no idea I had been left behind struggling. I thought for sure I'd have to call out to them. I didn't want to. It was at that moment I realized again how big I was. Somehow I managed to get my leg up and carefully pull myself up, but it wasn't easy. It was extremely difficult. When everyone opted to go through again, I opted out. I'd had enough.

During that same trip we decided to do some shopping. If you're familiar with St. George you know how hot it can get. We were there in the middle of July––the very hottest month. It was sweltering. We decided to take a break from the heat inside the air-conditioned shops and pick out new swimsuits while we were at it.

Inside Old Navy we each selected a number of cute tankinis to try on. While each of my friends found success, I found failure. None of them fit. Not even the XL. Not even remotely. I ended up buying a pair of men's size medium board shorts.

I paired it with an oversized tank and called it good. At that moment I felt frumpy in comparison to my friends.

So many experiences like that happened during the summer of 2007. Perhaps they had been happening all along, but by that summer I'd had enough. Each and every bad experience got under my skin like fingernails on a chalk board. I was tired of being the big friend. I was tired of people worrying whether I could complete things, participate in things, or fit into things. I was tired of being embarrassed about my body. I was tired of hiding from the camera. I was tired of being the friend who took all the pictures but never wanted to be in them. I was tired of trying to overcompensate by having great hair, makeup, and jewelry in order to feel better about myself. I was tired of feeling older than I was. I was tired. Period.

And I was done.

I think it was then that I had my breaking point. Everything came to a head. I was 37. I was ashamed I'd let most of my 30s go, and that somehow my body had gotten out of hand. 40 was right around the corner, and I wanted to do something about it.

> Unless I want my children to give up on their dreams, I can't give up on mine."
>
> – Liza Hughs, IFBB Fitness Pro

So when I ran into my friend at the craft store and she told me her husband could get me a great deal on a gym pass, I snagged it. It was one of those times when you act first and ask for permission later. I didn't want to talk with my husband first. I knew what he would say. I'd had gym memberships in the past and never followed through. I'd go at first but then stop. I'd find an excuse. I knew he wouldn't approve of me making the same mistake again. But somehow deep inside I knew this time would be different. It had to be. I felt it. I was compelled to change my body. So, I wrote her a check and did it. I signed up. I later told my husband, and he shook his head in disbelief. But it was too late.

I just knew this time I'd follow through.

The day Dakota started first grade I hit the gym. It was his first day, and it was my first day. The first several weeks I spent most of my time on the bike or walking on the treadmill. I'd been to the gym with my mom as a teenager, so I knew a bit about weight training, but not much. So instead, I spent my time doing cardio but observing what others were doing on the weight machines. I was a very good observer. When I was done with cardio, I'd mess around on the machines. I didn't know anything about form. I didn't know how heavy to go, how many sets, or how many reps. I didn't know which machines worked which body part. I didn't have a clue. But I toyed around on them just the same. I had every entitlement that everyone else there did. I pretended to know what I was doing. And when trainers (some of them being real salespeople with salesman-like attitudes) approached me to help (for a fee of course) I declined.

I did this for a couple of months. Cardio and machines. I made a habit of taking books with me to the gym to read. I read the entire Twilight series on the bike. I could get lost in my books while doing cardio. When I wasn't reading, I was

> The person
> who makes
> a success of
> living is the one
> who sees his
> goal steadily
> and aims for it
> unswervingly.
> That is
> dedication."
>
> – Cecil B. D. Mille

watching the trainers train. I had a few favorites. But there was one female trainer in particular I was impressed with. She was extremely athletic-looking and had the best arms. Her shoulders popped. She was cut. I wanted to look like her. There were other trainers there that looked like they knew what they were doing, but I wanted her to train me. I didn't want a guy. I wanted a girl who could relate to me, my body type, and the fun womanly issues we deal with. So, one morning I approached her. I simply told her I wanted her arms and that she needed to train me. She was a busy trainer. She had a lot of clients. She sized me up and said, "okay".

That was the beginning.

She was a figure competitor. When I approached her she had been cutting up for a show. She was lean. At that point I didn't even know what a figure competitor was.

Hiring a trainer when I first started was one of the best decisions I ever made. She took me around to several of the machines. She taught me about proper form. She taught me about drop sets. She gave me structure, a plan, and confidence. With her help I felt strong. I was well on my way.

By December I'd dropped 20 pounds. I was now roughly 150 pounds. I was back into a size 10, and I felt on top of the world. For the first time in years I felt attractive. I felt pretty. I loved that I had to go shopping to get smaller clothes. I loved giving away all my bigger clothes. I was happy to shop for trendy clothes and accessories. It almost felt like I was discovering a long-lost and forgotten me. It felt great!

Around that same time my trainer asked me if I had any interest in competing. She showed me her pictures and she told me I should try it. She realized that I was a hard worker and that I would follow through with every workout she gave me and then some. I could see some changes in my body without a doubt, but I'd never thought about competing. I felt I still had so much further to go. Apparently she saw something in me that I didn't see yet myself.

When I made the commitment to take my body back I also made a promise to myself to try everything. I started a bucket list and was adding goals to it daily. I no longer wanted my life to live me; I wanted to live my life. I wanted to take charge. I wanted to try new things. I wanted to have adventures. I wanted to grow old and have no regrets.

So when my trainer asked me about competing I figured why not? What could it hurt? At the very worst I might not be stage-ready by the time the competition came around, but I knew I would be so much further along than if I didn't have a goal. So I went for it on complete faith. I did not look the part, and a part of me was so embarrassed to even tell people what I was doing. What if I failed? What if I changed my mind? What if leaned out and didn't have any muscle? What if I was the laughing stock of the competition? What would people think? All of these thoughts ran through my mind. I was scared. But I was excited too. What if

I looked great? I decided to focus on the latter.

One year from the first day I set foot in that gym I competed in my first competition. I took 2nd in my first show. I couldn't have been more proud.

That year was eventful.

My bucket list continued to grow, and I made a point to compete in whatever I could.

That next March I ran my first 5k with several more to follow.

In May 2008 I competed in my first sprint triathlon, following with a second one in June.

In July 2008 I ran my first 10k with a second one later that month.

In September 2008 I stepped on stage for my first figure competition and participated in a second one in October.

In November 2008 I ran my first half marathon.

It became a year where my mottos became, "make it count," "never say never," and "giving up is not an option." It felt great.

Since then I've gone on to compete in seven shows, bringing home five trophies in the process. I've led

"You are never too old to set another goal or to dream a new dream."

– C.S. Lewis

my team two years in a row for the Wasatch Back Ragnar Relay. I've run four half marathons and two full marathons. Most recently I qualified for the Boston Marathon, which I'll be running in spring 2011.

In January I'll finally be 40—the age I've been dreading for the last three years. My mom competed in lightweight bodybuilding when she was 40. She has been and will always be my inspiration. I remember when I was 37––at my highest weight, unhappy, with bad experience piling upon bad experience—and I would think about my mom and how different our lives were. When she was 37 she looked amazing. When she was 40 she was at her peak. I wanted nothing more than to do the same.

One of my goals was to stand on the same stage my mom did when she competed. She competed in the Emerald Cup back in 1987. I stood on that same stage not just one year but two years in a row—with my proud parents in the crowd. It was a surreal experience. It is still run by the same people, and to date, it's been my favorite show experience.

My dad was a runner—and now I am.
My mom was a bodybuilder—and now I am.

I am so thankful for second chances. I feel like I am finally starting my life and living it the way that I really want to.

What I've learned is it's never too late. We all can improve. We all have it in us. It starts with perception, drive, and willpower. You have to want it bad enough. You have to make a series of right choices. And when you do fail, you need to get back up and push forward. Don't give up. Don't give in. Don't let bad habits and old lifestyles win. I can say this with confidence because I fought those demons too.

Looking forward I can't wait to celebrate my 40th birthday. That wasn't the case before. Now I plan my goals by thinking big––by looking at what bucket list items I want to accomplish next. The only difference between now and a few years ago is this: I know when I say I'll do something there is a really good chance I'll actually do it, and if not, I'll fail trying my hardest.

"People are always blaming their circumstances for what they are. I don't believe in circumstances. The people who really make it in this world are the ones who get up and look for the circumstances they want and if they can't find them, they make them."

– Unknown

MAKE ONE SMALL CHANGE

Make one small change. That's all I suggest. If you feel so inclined you might want to choose a couple, but do something. Eating clean and exercising doesn't initially have to be an all-or-nothing feat. You can make changes slowly, one at a time, until you feel you are making progress. Once you feel you have conquered that new change, try a new one, and then another one. It worked for me. In the list below you will find some of the real changes I slowly incorporated into my life as I struggled to lose weight and gain my life back. I didn't do them all at once. I'm sure I would have failed like I had time and time before had I tried to do that. Just one change made all the difference. Look through the list below and choose one. You can do this. Make one small change.

> Things that were hard to bear are sweet to remember."
>
> – Lucius Annaeus Seneca

Subscribe to everything

Newsletters, magazines, texts, books. When I first started losing weight, I'd spend countless hours on the bike, the treadmill, or the elliptical. I would get so bored. I found if I had something to read, the time would pass more quickly. I started subscribing to every health magazine imaginable. My passion started there but it didn't end there. I picked up some books at the store. I subscribed to my favorite sites online. I made sure that every time I turned around I was surrounded by information on running, weight training, anatomy, cooking, and fitness in general. I am still a student of fitness, and I still love to read up on everything. It hasn't changed.

Hang motivational quotes

On the fridge, on the mirror, in the car, and near the computer. I've done this ever since I was a kid. If I wanted something bad enough, I'd hang a picture of what I wanted. This time around if I heard a quote I liked or found a picture of someone who inspired me, I hung it up in places I'd see over and over. It helped keep me on track and focused.

It's hard to pull out the Ben & Jerry's with a picture of Jamie Eason on the outside of the freezer.

What is your motto?

I made my motto "Make it Count" each and every day. This was something personal to me. I suggest that you find your own motto, your own inspiration. "Make it Count" worked for me. Every day I told myself to "make it count." Whether I was at the gym, doing a cardio session, out for a run, or prepping food I soon discovered everything counts. You might as well make it work in a positive way. Maximum results can only come from maximum effort.

Change your mindset

Decide failure and giving up are no longer an option. I could count on two hands how many times I've tried to lose weight over the years. Up and down, up and down. After marrying my husband my weight never really went all the way back down to where it was when I was younger, but I still yo-yoed quite a bit. In the fall of 2007 I decided I had had enough. Something changed mentally. Giving up was no longer an option. Failure was not an option. I changed my mindset. Up to this moment I had always given up at some point and retreated to old habits. Then I would return to my old lifestyle. This time it was different, and it's because I didn't allow myself to turn back. When I speak with new friends who are on the same path hoping to lose weight, build muscle, or lean out, that's the single most important bit of advice I share with them. I really think the first commitment has to come within. Otherwise you can easily be distracted, discouraged, and give up. Not an option!

Switch from soda to something better.

I switched from Diet Pepsi to Propel. Sounds easy enough, right? I was a big Pepsi drinker. One time I tried Jenny Craig early in my 30s. The first week I dropped 8 pounds. Yeah, I changed my food that week, but the biggest change came from eliminating the soda. I honestly believe the soda bloated me and made me retain water (not to mention all the junk it was putting into my body). This time around when I eliminated Pepsi, I knew it was extremely important for me to find a substitute. I had to find something I liked equally as much that would fill that Pepsi void, and it couldn't be plain water. At the time I knew that wouldn't work for me. So, I found Propel. I kid you not: if you would have seen me back then every day for two straight years without fail I had a Propel bottle in my hand. Everywhere I went I had a Propel. I chugged it. I looked for sales. I stocked up. If I ran out, I filled it back up. I could have been a walking advertisement for that company. To give you an example, my neighbor's little girl one time was browsing through a magazine, and she told her mom, "Look mom, Jenny!" When she looked to see what she was referring to, she got a good chuckle when she realized her little girl was pointing to a Propel ad. That's how much I drank it. I knew as long as I had a full belly from Propel (water) I wouldn't be drinking soda. I also knew I wouldn't be snacking on junk.

Gum.

On that same note, gum has been a lifesaver for me. My favorite is Orbit Maui Melon Mint. No substitutes. I buy it by the carton, and I keep it in my food storage. Gum keeps my mouth busy. I like to eat, as I'm guessing you do, so gum fools my body. It tastes good, and as long as I am chewing, I'm not snacking.

During contest prep for shows I chew it literally all day long. It might not work for everyone, but it works for me, and it might just work for you!

Water.

Challenge yourself to drink a gallon of water every day by noon. Once I was in the habit of drinking Propel and not soda, I knew the next step was to increase my water intake. This is still a goal of mine today. I now buy water in 1-gallon jugs. Every day I try to drink at least 2/3 of it by noon. Most mornings I am at my computer––reading, checking my email, writing, watching the news, you name it. That's when I am still. It's a perfect time to have the water by my side where I can drink it––and quickly. If I don't, I end up sipping it through the day and never quite reaching my goal. Not to mention the fact that in the morning I am home, so if I need a bathroom, it's close by. If I try to chug it later in the day when I am running the kids around, finding a bathroom is not always the easiest thing to do!

Find snack alternatives.

Switch out empty-calorie snacks to protein shakes or something nutritious. I eat a variety of different snacks throughout the day, but they are all nutritious. Back in the day I'd have three large meals and then I'd snack on junk—candy, chips, excessive peanuts, cookies, whatever—in between. One of the easiest changes for me at the time was to drop the snacks and replace them with an all-in-one protein drink or shake. I'd have a shake in the morning pre-workout, breakfast, morning snack/shake, lunch, afternoon snack/shake, and then dinner. It helped me at the time. I don't recommend having three shakes a day long-term, but when I was trying to cut out the excess eating and snacking, it was something easy I could replace it with. I hadn't quite developed the talent of prepping my food in advance. I wanted convenience. That's what I was used to. I wanted immediate. Shakes provided that. Now I have several go to snacks that I rely on.

Stop buying white bread.

Bottom line: if white bread is in the house you're going to eat it. Same goes for pasta, muffins, etc. Either don't buy bread, or if you are going to, buy whole wheat, whole grain, or Ezekiel. Three years ago I had no clue what Ezekiel bread was, but I knew the difference between white and wheat, and I knew wheat was better. I'd read that mixed-grain wasn't necessarily as beneficial as whole-grain so I made more of an effort to only bring whole grains home. It's amazing thinking back at how breads and pastas made up a large part of my diet. I've slowly weaned myself off both, and I rarely have either one. I do love Ezekiel (sprouted grains), and I'll allow myself a treat every now and again, but the great thing is, I've found other foods I like equally as much that are so much more beneficial for my body. Now I don't even miss the breads and pastas. If it's a cheat meal, and we are at Texas Roadhouse BBQ, that's another story. Their rolls are amazing!!

"A man who wants something will find a way; a man who doesn't will find an excuse."

– Stephan Dolley Jr.

Be prepared before you go out.

Study the menus and nutritional information of your favorite restaurants and chose entrees ahead of time. This helped me to be more conscious about where I went when I went out. So much of our time is spent with friends and family in circumstances over which we have little control. I love date nights with my hubby and with my friends. There are so many wonderful restaurants, but most of the entrees found on the menus are unhealthy. They are laden with fats, too many carbs, and are over-salted. Whenever we go out I try to know the plan in advance. I want to know where we are going. That way I can start formulating a plan of what I am going to eat. I look up their menus online when possible. I review their nutritional information if they have it posted. At the restaurant, I'll ask for this information too. This might sound like a lot of trouble and might even be a little embarrassing at first, but knowledge is power. There are so many entrees I would have thought to be healthy, and later find they are just as bad as the rest of them. Making this choice is also empowering because it puts you in control of what you are taking into your body. I can think of a recent time when we went out to dinner with several other couples. We chose to eat at an Italian restaurant. First thought? Yum. Second thought? Holy cow, what am I going to eat there? To my husband's embarrassment I asked for a nutritional breakdown of their menu; they only had one on hand and didn't even know where to search for it. It took them around five minutes, but they did find it. While the others at the table were reviewing their menus, I was reviewing the nutritional sheet, and I made my choice based off of that. What's interesting is every singe person at the table wanted to see the nutritional breakdown once I was done. They were all curious to see how their choices measured up. It's worth the time and effort to plan. Some entrees have as many calories, fat, and carbs as your body needs for an entire day. Scary thought!

Start eating at home more and out less.

We were the king and queen of eating out several times a week. Even if we tried to eat at healthier places or make healthier choices, nothing compares to home-cooked clean-eating meals. At home I have complete control of what I cook, how I cook it, and how it's seasoned. It might not be the most convenient, but it's the most rewarding for the long term. It stems back to planning and trying new things. Now I love to cook. I try new recipes all the time. Many times when we do go out I am disappointed, knowing that at home I could make it better. I didn't always feel that way though, and it does take some discipline in the kitchen. All I know is I like the scale a lot more when we are eating at home.

You are in charge.

Allow yourself to be picky when ordering in restaurants. There is absolutely nothing wrong about asking for food to be done a certain way. You are the customer, and you are paying for your meal. If you want to know how something is

"I do today what you won't, so I can do tomorrow what you can't."

– Unknown

prepared, ask. If you want it prepared differently, ask. If you want something on the side or not at all, ask. That is the job of being an informed customer, and it is their job as a helpful server. As long as you ask tactfully and with respect, I think it's perfectly appropriate to have your order cooked the way you like it. I used to laugh at one of my friends in particular who took five minutes to order her dinner. I judged her prematurely. Now I'm that person. But I am okay with that.

Prepare food ahead of time.

This takes time and it might take a while to build it in to a habit, but it really is worth it. Plan your week. Buy your meats, fruits, veggies, grains, everything. Then give yourself a couple of hours to chop, slice, prep, and cube your food for the week. Store everything in sealed containers for easy access. When I get the munchies I go straight for the fridge. Don't we all? We are programmed to get food when hungry from the pantry or the fridge. If you don't have healthy options to choose from, you'll go for the junk. No one wants to wait around to prepare an elaborate meal or even a snack when hungry. That's why it's so important to have a plan and healthy options readily available when you need them. Have green salads, cooked chicken, broiled flank, tuna salads, hardboiled eggs, sliced fruit, clean veggies--you just need options. That's the key.

Study the trainers at the gym.

Over the years I've worked with a number of different trainers. I'd signed up with trainers before, but I always got "stuck" with whomever's turn it was to have a new customer. Even with as little as I knew then I often felt I knew more than they did. It was hard for me, a 30-something-year-old to take direction from an indecisive 20-year-old. I often failed the trainers because I felt they failed me.

In 2007 when I started back to gym with a new determination, many trainers approached me. I resisted. Instead, I held back and I watched them. I watched how they worked with their clients. I studied the exercises they did. I evaluated everything. Then, when I was ready, I approached the trainer I wanted to work with. I chose her. I didn't allow the trainer to choose me. My first trainer, LuAnn, who is now one of my closest friends, had the most amazing arms. She was "buff," for lack of a better term. I chose her. My pick-up line? "I want your arms. You need to train me." You may or may not want a trainer, but even if you don't, there is so much to be learned by studying one. You can learn new exercises, study their form, the order in which they do exercises, sets, reps, etc. Trainers are an invaluable tool.

Don't be afraid to lift weights.

I talk to and read about women all the time who are afraid to lift weights. I hear excuse after excuse: "I don't want to work out in there...the guys are in there." "I don't know what to do, and I don't want to look like an idiot." "I don't want to get bulky." "I've lifted before, and I didn't see any difference, so why even do it?" Regardless of the excuse, weight training is an important tool in losing weight, toning up, and reshaping the body. I knew that. I knew I had to do it. I also knew that I would look a little silly as I got started. Just the same, it was an essential tool in helping me get to where I am today. As I mentioned before, I studied people. I studied trainers. I watched what they did, and then I imitated them. With time I grew more confident. With time I saw results. With time I added on. It took the first step though of just doing it--regardless of how I looked or what people thought.

Set a goal.

As a teenager I was a goal-setter. I knew what I wanted. I went after everything with passion and vigor. If I wanted it, I attacked it with every fiber in me. Student Council, FBLA, drill team, Jazz Choir, sports, boys. If I wanted it, I set a goal and I figured out a way to accomplish it. Then, during my 20s and most of my 30s those goals subsided. Rather than living my life, my life lived me. I had some great experiences in spite of my lack of direction, but I don't believe I accomplished nearly what I could have had I actually set goals. Then in the fall of 2007 when I decided to lose weight and get fit, I reintroduced myself to the joy of goal making. I wasn't a runner when I first started, but I set a goal to run a 5k. I did this with a friend. I felt like a complete fool, because I really was not a runner by any stretch of the imagination. I felt old, uncoordinated, and winded every time I hit the pavement. Wait, I hadn't even hit the pavement at that point. All of my jogging had been done on the treadmill. What was I doing running a race? But I did it. We did it. And somewhere along the way of training I found my joy in running. The race itself sealed the deal. I loved the environment. I loved the excitement. I loved being youthful just by participating. I loved every part of it. All because I set a goal—even if at the time it was a lofty one.

Start reading labels.

Again, reflecting back on my Jenny Craig and Weight Watchers days, I remember the importance of reading labels. They mentioned that a number of times. Nutritional information was stressed in every class, and in all the literature. I never quite got the knack for interpreting the labels the way they wanted me to, but I did start reading them. Now I read the label every time I set foot in the grocery store or pull something out of the pantry. I check the calories, fats, carbs, protein, and sodium. After a few years of practice, I learned what was high, moderate, or low. Sometimes I'm shocked, so I quickly put whatever it is back on the shelf. No two brands are created the same. Every manufacturer creates their recipes just a bit different. To give you an example, when I first tried Greek Yogurt I was startled to find that two similar sized Greek Yogurts (different manufacturers) had completely different protein amounts. One had around 13 grams of protein while the other had around 24 grams of protein. That's a fairly significant difference. The same goes for sodium. I love to include tuna in my diet, and I love the tuna packets I can throw in my purse. However, the sodium in packaged tuna is unreal. Recently one of the brands introduced low-sodium tuna packets. It's a fraction of what the normal sodium levels are in the competitors. With no hesitation I depleted their entire stock of low-sodium tuna, knowing I would get enough sodium from all of the other foods in my diet. Check labels—it's totally worth it.

THE IMPORTANCE OF BREAKFAST

My mom used to tell me, "Breakfast is the most important meal of the day." I hated that. I'd get up early in the morning to finish my homework and I'd be in such a hurry, I rarely had time to get something down. Breakfast? Who had time for breakfast? I thought she just told me that to trick me into having breakfast. I didn't think there was any reasoning to back it up.

In my 20s, I skipped breakfast because I could. It was a challenge. I figured if I ate less in the morning when I wasn't hungry, I could eat more later. I was saving myself extra calories, right? I'd skip breakfast and make up for it at lunch or end up snacking on junk food by mid-morning. So really, skipping breakfast defeated the purpose of the good I thought I was trying to do.

In my 30s I started eating breakfast. I ate whatever I wanted. By my 30s I'd started gaining unwanted weight. So, why not eat breakfast? I really paid little attention to what I was eating. We'd stock up on bulk cereal, buying whatever sounded good for the best price. Sugary cereals weren't doing my figure any favors.

> "The principle is competing against yourself. It's about self-improvement, about being better than you were the day before."
>
> – Steve Young

It wasn't until I started training that I truly took the time to understand the importance of a proper breakfast.

You need breakfast for a number of reasons, but for the purpose of this book, let me just touch on a few.

First of all, it's not called "breakfast" for nothing. In the morning you are meant to break your fast-- meaning you need to fuel your body. You need food—not only to satisfy your hunger, but also to restore your glycogen stores. What does that mean? It's simply to give you energy. It utilizes all the remaining available energy. You need to refuel so that you don't feel fatigued. Even if you don't feel like you're running on empty first thing in the morning, by lunchtime you're likely to feel tired.

Second, you need breakfast to maintain focus and clarity. Think of a time when you've skipped breakfast. I know I, for one, become very irritable when I don't eat when I am supposed to. I become grumpy, and it's difficult for me to focus on anything until I've had something to eat. I can't think straight, my mind wanders, I'm anxious, and I can't sit still. Basically, when I haven't eaten, I'm good for nothing. The same goes for breakfast. In order to think clearly you need to start your day with a decent breakfast.

Third, having breakfast will help you make positive food choices all day long. It's true. I'm not saying that you'll always make healthy food choices, but a proper breakfast will help. By filling up with a good breakfast, you'll be less likely to give in to temptations later in the day. By making right choices early, you'll be more equipped to say no to temptations that come your way. And we all know sometimes temptations come in the strangest forms. It's not always cookies and ice cream. When you're hungry temptation comes in whatever's handy and convenient.

While I don't suggest you skip any meal, the one you definitely shouldn't skip is breakfast.

And for me personally? I can't think of a better breakfast than oatmeal.

WHY OATMEAL?

For as long as I can remember I've always had some form of oatmeal for breakfast.

As a kid I pounded the sugary instant oatmeal packages. I'd eat two or three at a time, and I especially loved Peaches and Cream. That was by far my breakfast of choice during Elementary School. I remember I used to leave the maple and brown sugar ones for last; they were my least favorite.

Then as a teenager I had it in a different form. As a family we'd head up to Whistler to ski. My loft was open, and I'd wake up every morning before a full day of skiing to mom cooking oatmeal on the stove. I can still remember the smell. If any of us would complain about having oatmeal again, mom would quickly remind us, "You're having oatmeal because it sticks to the ribs." I can't even count how many times I heard that. Now I think how much mom would have loved having an overnight Crockpot oatmeal recipe. It would have saved her so much time.

It wasn't until I began competing that oatmeal would play another important role in my diet. Oatmeal and oats quickly found a permanent place on every update of my diet regardless of which trainer I worked with. Since I started competing I've had the opportunity to work with some world-class trainers and each one of them always included oats in some fashion on my daily meal plan.

It wasn't until I started competing that Sandy, one of my trainers, introduced me to what would become a favorite snack—dry oats mixed with sugar substitute and cinnamon. I take this everywhere: on road trips, to the pool, on vacation, to the movies—you name it. I even started including it as a pre-race ritual. I quickly got several of my friends eating it too. This little snack keeps my mouth busy and happy. As long as I am chewing on dried oats I'm not snacking on movie popcorn, road trip chips, poolside snacks, and fast-food junk. It really has saved me more times than I can count. And even though I am loading up on extra carbs, they are good carbs.

After adding oatmeal as a continual staple in my diet I began to get antsy. I wanted a change. I wanted more flavor. I wanted to try oatmeal in new and more creative ways. Being a happy homemaker, I had time to spare. I could try new things, knowing that by trial and error I'd find some successes. I craved new oatmeal recipes.

And that's when my true obsession with oatmeal began.

I tried the basics: simply adding things to my stovetop cooked oatmeal. Then I tried Crockpot oatmeal, overnight oatmeal, and then finally my favorite, baked oatmeal.

Oats have so many health benefits too––more than I can list here––but the ones I've read time and time again are worth repeating.

Here are the top ten reasons I eat oatmeal:

1. Research has shown the heart benefits of eating oatmeal daily. In fact, more than 40 studies show that eating **oatmeal may help reduce the risk of heart disease and lower cholesterol.** Quaker suggests that all it takes is ¾ cup of oatmeal each day to help lower cholesterol. The soluble fiber in oats can help maintain the good cholesterol your body needs, while helping to remove LDL or "bad" cholesterol. The Food and Drug Administration announced that oatmeal could carry a label claiming it may reduce the risk of heart disease when combined with a low-fat diet.

2. Oatmeal can help control your weight by helping you feel full longer. This is because the soluble fiber in oatmeal absorbs a considerable amount of water, which can significantly slow down the digestive process.

3. **Oats are easy to use and easy to find.** In fact, it has been estimated that eighty percent of U.S. households currently have oats in their kitchen cupboards.

4. Because the soluble fiber in oats can help to control blood glucose levels, new research suggests that eating **oatmeal may reduce the risk for type 2 diabetes.**

5. **Oats are 100% natural.** With the exception of certain flavored varieties, if you look at the ingredients on a canister of rolled oats, you will usually find only one ingredient: rolled oats.

6. Recent studies have shown that a diet that includes **oatmeal may help reduce high blood pressure.** The soluble fiber provided by oatmeal is linked to the reduction. Oats contain more soluble fiber than whole wheat, rice or corn.

7. Oatmeal is a good source of protein, complex carbohydrates and iron and also **contains a wide array of vitamins, minerals and antioxidants.**

8. The fiber and other nutrients oatmeal contains **may reduce the risk for certain cancers.**

9. **Oatmeal is quick and convenient.** Most oatmeal can be cooked within 10 minutes. Heartier baked oatmeal can be prepared in under 10 minutes and cooked within 30.

10. **Oatmeal can be absolutely delicious!** Whether instant, cooked on the stove or baked in the oven, all you need is imagination to come up with the combination of flavors you can fit into a serving of oatmeal.
(For more info see MrBreakfast.com)

I'm still trying new recipes all the time. I haven't stopped looking, and I haven't stopped creating. As long as I can buy oats in bulk I'll be trying new ways to put my own spin on cooking oatmeal.

Happy fixins and make something good!

WHAT'S IN MY FRIDGE AND IN MY PANTRY

Jenny's Shopping List

Oats:

Old-Fashioned

Quick

Steel cut oats

Oatmeal Alternatives (such as brown rice, quinoa, grits, and creamed rice)

Individual Serving Baking Dish – This can be purchased at Wal Mart, Target, or online. Ramekins come in all sizes and are approximately $2.00 per bowl.

These items can be purchased at Costco, a supermarket or a health food store:

Quinoa

Flaxseed

Almond Milk

Brown rice (such as cinnamon, ginger, nutmeg, apple pice spice, pumpkin pie spice, citris zest, etc.)

Nonfat cottage cheese

Greek yogurt

Fresh and frozen fruit

Spices

Dried fruits such as chopped dates, prunes, figs, etc.

Capella Drops – www.capellaflavordrops.com is the best source

Torani Syrups – www.torani.com and limited supply in most larger supermarkets and coffee specialty shops

MY FAVORITE PRODUCTS & WHERE TO FIND THEM

Torani Syrups

www.torani.com

Description: With the great flavors of Torani in your home, every drink and meal you make can be inspired. Their flavors range from citrus and berry to spicy and nutty.

Capella Flavors Inc.

www.capellaflavordrops.com

Description: Capella Drops are a water-soluble, highly concentrated multi-purpose flavoring. Flavor drops have a wide range of uses: protein shakes, smoothies, baked goods, water, etc.

TopForm Nutrition Supplements

www.mytopform.com

Description: As experienced health and fitness professionals, we recognize the need for a source of high-quality vitamins and nutritional supplements, and understand the importance for all-natural products that will not harm you or add undue stress to your system. TopForm Supplements manufacture and maintain their products to ensure quality and strength.

Sweetleaf Liquid Stevia Flavors

www.stevia.com

Description: SweetLeaf Liquid Stevia with all-natural flavors is convenient and easy to use.

ZERO calories. ZERO carbohydrates. ZERO glycemic index.
- Convenient and economical to use
- Only pennies per drop at retail
- Zero calories, carbs, and glycemic index
- A proprietary blend of all natural flavors
- Can be used in almost anything
- Great for cooking and baking

PB2 and FitNutz Powdered Peanut Butter

www.bellplantation.com

Description: Both companies offer an excellent tasting variety of peanut butter powders. At a fraction of the calories and fats of regular peanut butter you can enjoy that much more.

Nature's Hollow

www.natureshollow.com

Description: Nature's Hollow offers sugar-free jam, sugar-free syrup, sugar-free low-carb tomato homemade ketchup, and a sugar-free honey product. They use a great-tasting and good-for-you sweetener called Xylitol. Their sugar-free fruit preserves are all low in carbs and perfect for the diabetic and weight-conscious individual.

Navitas Naturals

www.navitasnaturals.com

Description: Nutrient-rich whole foods are best produced using organic agricultural methods with minimal processing. Focusing on both food safety and nutrition, they handle our premium superfoods with care. This includes third-party testing for all our products.

Voskos Greek Yogurt

www.voskos.com

Description: Organically and naturally delicious. It's nature's perfect superfood that may help prevent diseases and boost your immune and digestive system while you savor every creamy spoonful.

MY LIFE THEN & MY LIFE NOW

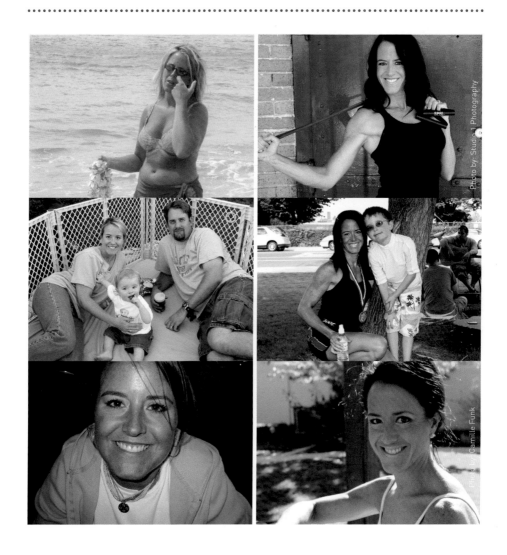

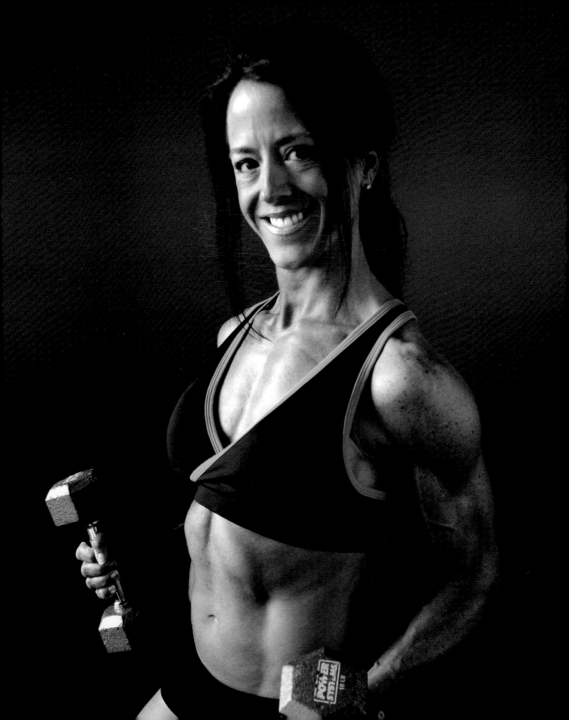

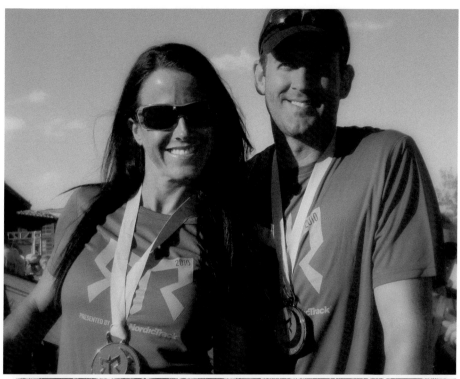

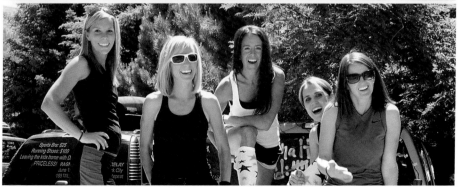

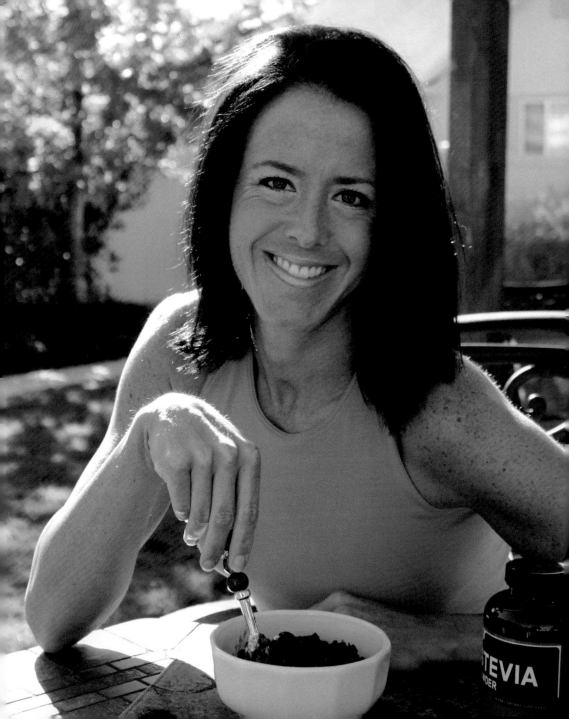

THE HEALTH BENEFITS OF EATING CLEAN

What does it mean to eat clean? Mostly it means avoiding foods that are packaged or contain preservatives. Clean foods are whole, natural foods like fruits and veggies, lean proteins, and complex carbohydrates. This includes foods like oatmeal, flax seed, dried fruits, and nuts. Things you want to avoid are white bread, hydrogenated fats, and refined sugar. Someone who is trying to eat clean cooks healthy meals, eliminates refined sugar, drinks a lot of water, and eats five to six small meals a day. Some clean foods you'll find extensively in this cookbook are:

Oat Groats and Steel Cut Oats.

Oat groats and steel cut oats are typically the best bet. Honestly, I wouldn't know an oat grout to save my life, but I'm very familiar with steel cut oats and use them frequently when cooking breakfast. Both are whole-grains chopped into smaller pieces, so maintain most of their nutritional value. They are higher in fiber, include more cholesterol lowering soluble fiber, take longer to digest, and help make you feel fuller longer! Since they are thicker when cooked, they tend to be chewier than traditional oatmeal, and they do take more time to cook as well. Plan on upwards of 30 minutes too cook either one! Steel cut oats can be found in most supermarkets and health food stores.

Old-fashioned Oatmeal.

If you choose not to have groats or steel cut oats the next best thing is old-fashioned oatmeal. This is what captured my heart. I'm a huge fan of old-fashioned oats and would eat them all day long for every meal if I could get away with it. Old-fashioned oats are first steamed to soften them, and then they are run through mills to flatten them. Some nutrients are lost in this process. Just the same, they are absolutely delicious and a real favorite of mine. Old-fashioned oats typically take 5-10 minutes to cook. Old-fashioned oats can be found just about anywhere, but I find the best pricing is when I buy in bulk at large wholesales like Costco.

Quick Oats.

Quick oats under go the same process as old-fashioned, but after they are rolled thin, they are cooked and dried again – losing even more of their important and beneficial nutrients. I very rarely cook with these any more – not when their alternatives are so much better! Quick oats usually only take a few minutes too cook. Like old-fashioned oats, quick oats can be found in most any grocery store.

Brown Rice.

The reason I cook with brown rice instead of white rice is because brown rice still maintains most of it's beneficial make-up. With brown rice only the outer hull is removed. With white rice, not only is the outer hull removed but the bran and most of the germ layer are also removed. After the entire process only a refined starch is left behind and contains only a fraction of its original counterpart. Brown rice may take a little longer to cook and may be a little nuttier tasting, but it has oodles more nutrition than white rice. Health benefits include lowering cholesterol and increased fiber. Brown rice typically takes an average of 40 minutes to cook. Brown rice can be found in any supermarket.

Quinoa.

I'm using quinoa more and more. One thing I found interesting about quinoa is it's not actually a grain but more of a seed, related to leafy green veggies like spinach and swiss chard. Quinoa is rich in proteins, nutty in flavor, available at most health food stores and only takes around 15-20 minutes to cook.

Apples.

Can protect against osteoporosis, protect against free-radical damage, lower cholesterol, and prevent cancer.

Peaches.

Keep the skin healthy, prevent cancer, are a good source of dietary fiber, have excellent antioxidant activity, and have sedative properties.

Raspberries.

Can help prevent cancer, protect the skin, can help keep the metabolic rate high, and also contain strong antioxidants.

Cinnamon.

Can help lower blood pressure and prevent cell damage. It has been shown to reduce blood glucose, and lower cholesterol.

Rhubarb.

May help to destroy cancer cells, helps to lower cholesterol, and has natural laxative properties.

Bananas

Are a great source of natural energy. Rich in potassium, they can reduce strokes and regulate blood pressure. The tryptophan in bananas can help the mind relax. Bananas can also help to restore and maintain regular bowel functions.

Almonds.

Can promote lower cholesterol levels, prevent heart disease and help with weight loss.

Strawberries.

Can help fight cancer, neutralize the effect of free radicals, lower high blood pressure and prevent heart disease. They also have anti-inflammatory properties.

Pineapples.

Are anti-inflammatory, aid in digestion, are high in anti-oxidants, and fight against free radicals.

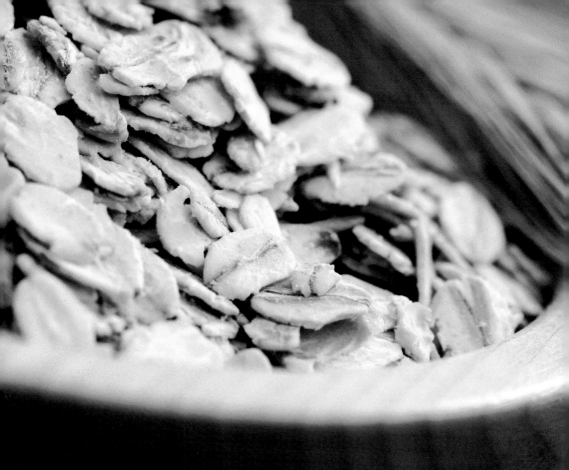

OATMEAL
RECIPES

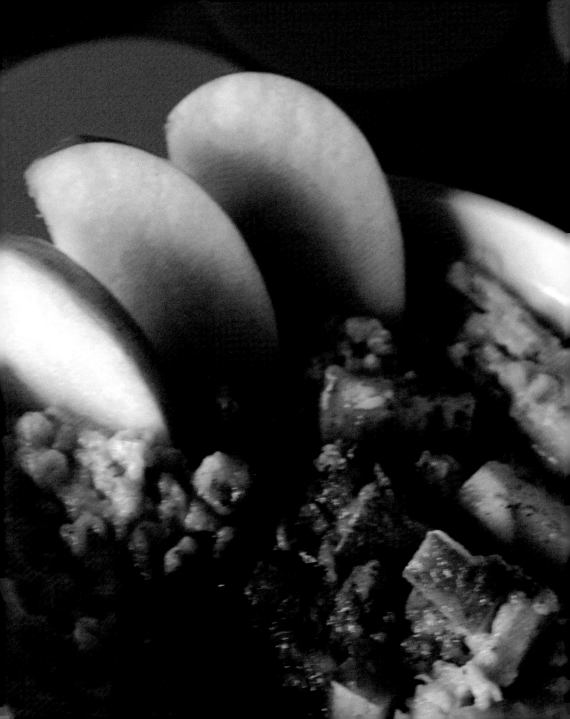

BAKED APPLE PIE OATMEAL

INGREDIENTS:

½ cup old-fashioned oats
1 cup water
2 egg whites
¼ tsp baking powder
pinch salt
¼ cup chopped apples
1 Tbsp golden raisins
pinch cinnamon
pinch apple pie spice
sugar substitute, to taste
½ tsp vanilla
1 Tbsp unsweetened almond milk
1 tsp brown sugar

DIRECTIONS:

Mix all but last two ingredients
and bake at 350 degrees for
30 minutes.
TIP: Add a pinch of brown sugar
and drizzle with almond milk.

Serving: 1
Prep Time: 3 minutes
Cooking Time: 30 minutes

One of my favorite memories is of when I was a little girl we'd go to
Grandma and Grandpa Passeys for Christmas. We lived in Washington while
Grandma and Grandpa lived in Utah, so it was quite the drive. After driving
for 17 hours straight and being absolutely dead tired, I remember the sweet
smell of Grandma's homemade apple pie the minute I stepped in the front
door. It somehow made the nightmare of the drive forgettable.

NUTRITION:

Calories 227 | Fat 3g | Sodium 52.5mg | Carbs 43.16g | Fiber 6.36g
Sugars 14.81g | Protein 8.69g

BAKED BANANA OATMEAL IN RUM

INGREDIENTS:

½ cup old-fashioned oats

¼ tsp baking powder

¼ tsp rum extract

¼ tsp vanilla

¼ tsp butter imitation butter
   (found in baking aisle)

1 cup water

sugar substitute, to taste

½ cup sliced banana

1 Tbsp almond slivers

2 egg whites

DIRECTIONS:

Combine in an oven-proof bowl and bake at 350 degrees for 30 minutes.

Serving: 1
Prep Time: 3 minutes
Cook Time: 30 minutes

By choice I don't drink, but I still love the flavoring a little imitation rum adds to desserts and breads – and this baked oatmeal.

NUTRITION:

Calories 269 | Fat 7g | Sodium 50mg | Carbs 43.3g | Fiber 6.8g
Sugars 12.4g | Protein 10.75g

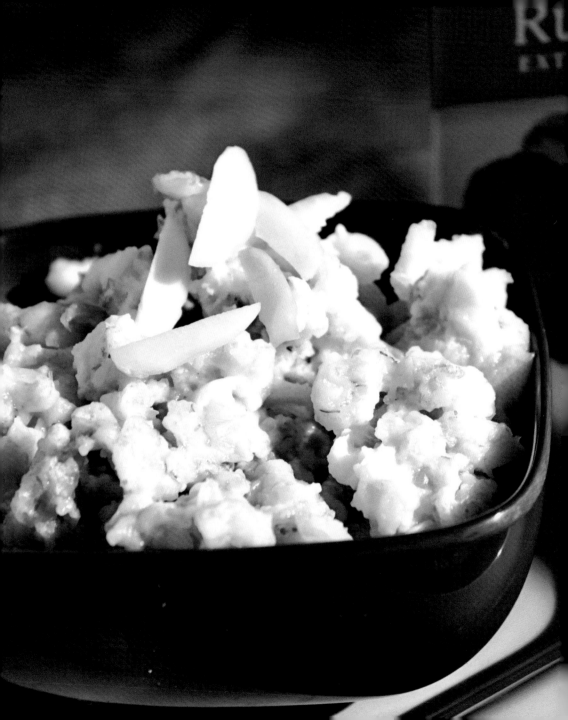

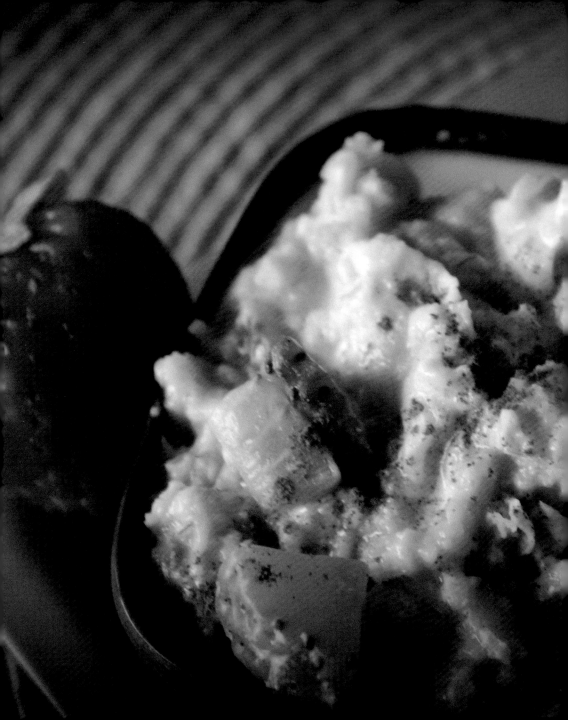

TART STRAWBERRY RHUBARB BAKED OATMEAL

INGREDIENTS:

½ cup old-fashioned oats

1 cup water

¼ tsp baking powder

¼ tsp cinnamon

¼ tsp imitation butter
   (found in baking aisle)

½ tsp vanilla

¼ cup sliced rhubarb

4-5 medium strawberries, sliced

2 egg whites

sugar substitute, to taste

DIRECTIONS:

Mix in an oven-proof bowl and bake at 350 degrees for 30 minutes.

Serving: 1
Prep Time: 3 minutes
Cook Time: 30 minutes

Growing up I remember Grandma Ward's Strawberry Rhubarb Pie. I loved it. Only Grandma made it. I haven't had Strawberry Rhubarb Pie in years. When I saw rhubarb in the grocery store, I knew I needed to try it in my oatmeal. I was pleasantly surprised at how good it tasted. A little more tart than my other oatmeal recipes, it still has the subtle sweetness from the strawberries.

NUTRITION:

Calories 175 | Fat 3.05g | Sodium 50.75mg | Carbohydrate 29.76g | Fiber 4.81g
Sugars 2.07g | Protein 8.5g

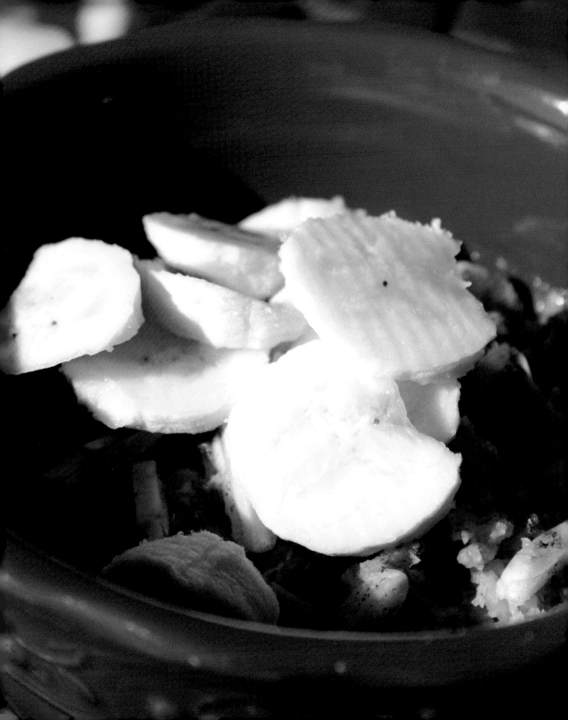

BANANA BREAD BAKED OATMEAL

INGREDIENTS:

½ banana

½ cup old-fashioned oats

1 cup water

3 Tbsp egg whites

2 Tbsp sugar-free Torani
    English Toffee syrup

sugar substitute, to taste

6 large walnut halves, broken

¼ tsp baking powder

DIRECTIONS:

Mash banana. Mix with other
ingredients in an oven-proof
bowl. Bake at 350 degrees
for 30 minutes.

Serving: 1

Prep Time: 3 minutes

Cook Time: 30 minutes

Bananas have gotten a bad rap. I love them. I think in small doses they can
be a great addition to breakfast—especially when your body is so hungry for
carbs. After a hard workout or a long run, this always hits the spot! Besides, I
have yet to meet a gal who doesn't crave banana bread.

NUTRITION:

Calories 232 | Fat 4.2g | Sodium 60.04mg | Carbs 42.01g | Fiber 6.13g | Sugars 11.8g

BANANA BREAD CROCKPOT STEEL CUT OATS

INGREDIENTS:

1 cup steel cut oats

4 cups water

1 tsp cinnamon

¼ cup brown sugar/
   Splenda blend

1 tsp vanilla

1 apple, peeled and diced

½ cup raisins

½ banana, sliced

¼ cup chopped walnuts

DIRECTIONS:

Coat the inside of your Crockpot first with cooking spray. Add all ingredients except for banana and walnuts. Mix well. Cover and cook on low for 8 hours. In the morning cut in banana and walnuts and serve. Top with a little almond milk, honey, or agave!

Serving: 4
Prep Time: 5 minutes
Cook Time: 6-7 hours on low

I love banana bread and if it's healthy, even better. For mornings when you're in a rush, this is a great go-to breakfast that's ready when you are.

NUTRITION:

Calories 256 | Fat 6g | Carbs 4g | Fiber 4g | Protein 4g

BROWN SUGAR AND BAKED DATE OATMEAL

INGREDIENTS:

½ cup old-fashioned oats

5 tsp nonfat cottage cheese

¼ tsp baking powder

sugar substitute, to taste

2 Tbsp Torani sugar-free Brown Sugar and Cinnamon syrup

½ tsp vanilla

28g chopped dates *(weighing the dates is easiest)*

1 cup water

dash cinnamon

DIRECTIONS:

Mix in an oven-proof bowl. Bake at 350 degrees for 30 minutes.

TIP: Try health food stores like Whole Foods or Good Earth when buying your favorite dried fruits in bulk. I bought the oat-covered chopped dates used in this recipe at Good Earth. I love them so much more than the ones prepackaged.

Serving: 4
Prep Time: 3 minutes
Cook Time: 30 minutes

It's no secret I love baked oatmeal, but when I first created this one, I had a hard time convincing myself to try new ones.

NUTRITION:

Calories 218 | Fat 3g | Sodium 74.88mg | Carbs 44.21g | Fiber 5.47g
Sugars 15.34g | Protein 7.7g

BLACK FOREST BAKED OATMEAL

INGREDIENTS:

½ cup old-fashioned oats

1 cup water

sugar substitute, to taste

¼ tsp baking powder

2 Tbsp Torani Dark Cherry
    sugar-free syrup

8 cherries, pitted and sliced

1 tsp unsweetened cocoa powder

2 egg whites

DIRECTIONS:

Mix in an oven-proof bowl
and bake at 350 degrees for
30 minutes.

Serving: 1

Prep Time: 5 minutes

Cook Time: 30 minutes

I'm 50% German, so my mom introduced me to the combination of cherries
with dark chocolate at a very young age. I remember one of my birthday cakes
in particular – it was a homemade Black Forest Cake compliments of mom.

NUTRITION:

Calories 194 | Fat 3.24g | Sodium 65mg | Carbs 33.85g | Protein 8.63g

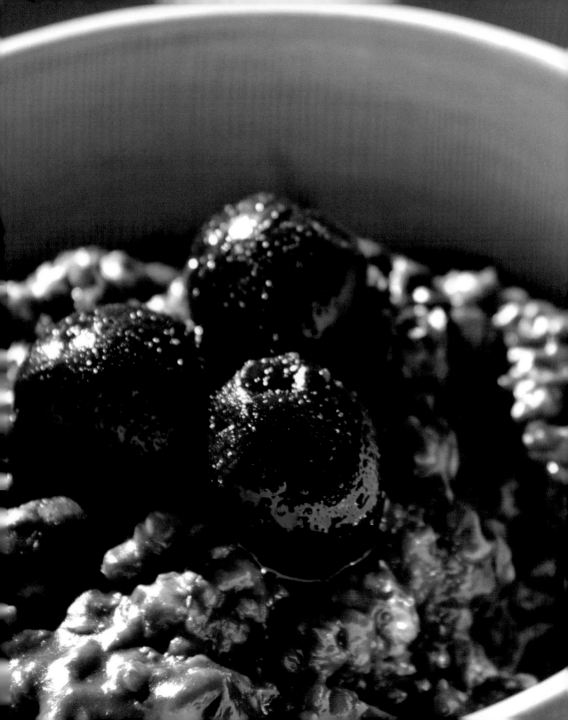

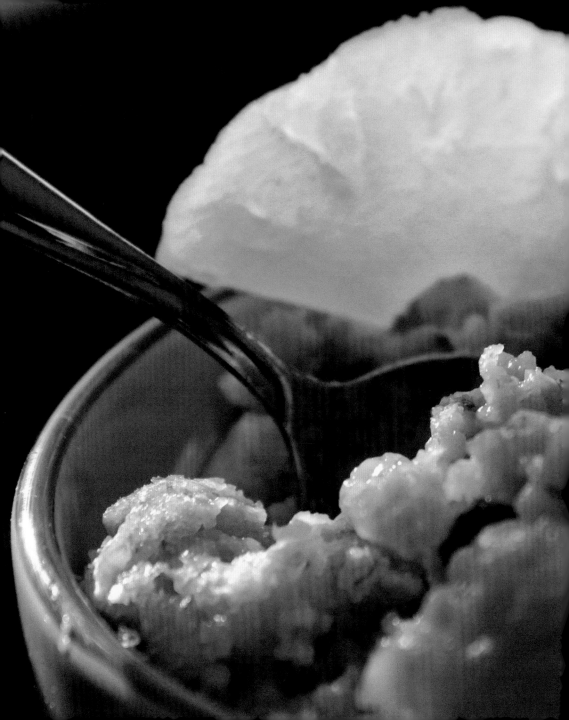

BROWN SUGAR PINEAPPLE BAKED OATMEAL

INGREDIENTS:

½ cup old-fashioned oats

1 cup water

¼ tsp baking powder

1 oz. dried pineapple

2 Tbsp sugar-free Torani Brown
  Sugar Cinnamon syrup

1 tsp raisins

sugar substitute, to taste

pinch brown sugar

almond milk, to taste

DIRECTIONS:

Mix all ingredients with the exception of the brown sugar in an oven-proof bowl. Bake at 350 degrees for 30 minutes. Remove oatmeal from oven and sprinkle small amount of brown sugar on top. Increase oven temp to broil. Return oatmeal to the oven and broil for 2-3 more minutes. Remove again. Drizzle with almond milk.

Serving: 1
Prep Time: 3 minutes
Cook Time: 30 minutes

This is another one of my favorites. It seems like it's not a summer potluck if someone doesn't bring the pineapple upside-down cake. This oatmeal's flavor and texture take me to summer in a good way. Just need the maraschino cherry!

NUTRITION:

Calories 265 | Fat 4g | Sodium 59.12mg | Carbs 49.72g | Fiber 5.22g
Sugars 20.5g | Protein 8.36g

CHOCOLATE-DRIZZLED PB TOFFEE BAKED OATMEAL

INGREDIENTS:

⅓ cup old-fashioned oats

⅛ tsp baking powder

2 Tbsp Torani sugar-free English Toffee syrup

1 tsp PB2 powder

sugar substitute, to taste

⅔ cup water

5 tsp nonfat cottage cheese

1 Tbsp Walden Farms 0 cal chocolate sauce

From time to time fruit just won't do?.

DIRECTIONS:

Mix all but the last ingredient in an oven-proof bowl and bake at 350 degrees for 30 minutes. When done, drizzle with Walden Farms Zero Calorie Chocolate Sauce.

Serving: 1
Prep Time: 3 minutes
Cook Time: 30 minutes

NUTRITION:

Calories 137 | Fat 2.75g | Sodium 139.38mg | Carbs 21.52g | Fiber 3.66g
Sugars 1.79g | Protein 8.53g

CARAMEL APPLE PIE OATMEAL

INGREDIENTS:

½ cup old-fashioned oats

1 cup water

2 egg whites

2 Tbsp unsweetened organic
    applesauce

⅓ apple, sliced

1 Tbsp raisins

¼ tsp baking powder

sugar substitute, to taste

dash cinnamon

2 Tbsp sugar-free Torani
    Caramel syrup

DIRECTIONS:

Mix ingredients in an oven-proof
bowl. Bake at 350 degrees
for 30 minutes.

Serving: 1
Prep Time: 3 minutes
Cook Time: 30 minutes

Another favorite treat of mine is caramel apples – especially from Rocky
Mountain Chocolate Factory. I justify them by telling myself the fruit is healthy.
Ha! This is one caramel apple that really IS healthy.

NUTRITION:

Calories 250 | Fat 3g | Sodium 59.61mg | Carbs 48.74g | Fiber 6.84g
Sugars 19.66g | Protein 8.75g

DIRTY CHAI BAKED OATMEAL

INGREDIENTS:

½ cup old-fashioned oats

1 cup water

¼ tsp baking powder

2 egg whites

1 Tbsp instant coffee or sugar-free Torani Coffee syrup

2 tsp Big Train low-carb chai mix

sugar substitute, to taste

DIRECTIONS:

Mix the above. Place in oven-proof dish and bake at 350 degrees for 30 minutes. Drizzle with unsweetened almond milk.

Serving: 1
Prep Time: 3 minutes
Cook Time: 30 minutes

Growing up near Seattle, I was in the Mecca for good coffee. I grew up loving the smell and as a teenager drank lattes daily. Back then I didn't know about nor did I care about calories, sugars, and fat. I ordered full-fat sugary lattes and enjoyed every sip. Then chai came along... I had to create a recipe that would have the same flavor as the real thing without all the unnecessary calories and fats. Mission accomplished.

NUTRITION:

Calories 201 | Fat 4.48g | Sodium 103.37mg | Carbs 33.77g | Fiber 4g
Sugars 2.44g | Protein 8.84g

DARK CHERRY BAKED OATMEAL

INGREDIENTS:

½ cup old-fashioned oats

1 cup water

¼ tsp baking powder

3 Tbsp Torani sugar-free Dark
  Cherry Syrup

2 egg whites

Sugar substitute, to taste

8 fresh cherries, pitted and sliced

DIRECTIONS:

Mix in an oven-proof dish. Bake at
350 degrees for 30 minutes.

Serving: 1
Prep Time: 5 minutes
Cook Time: 30 minutes

This is especially good when fresh Bing cherries are in season.

NUTRITION:

Calories 188 | Fat 3.08g | Sodium 112.5mg | Carbs 33.35g | Protein 8.63g

DRIED CRANBERRY BAKED OATMEAL

INGREDIENTS:

½ cup old-fashioned oats

¼ tsp ground cinnamon

¼ tsp baking powder

¼ tsp almond extract

dash salt

½ cup water

½ cup unsweetened almond milk

2 egg whites

½ tsp vanilla

2 Tbsp dried cranberries

spray butter

dash brown sugar

DIRECTIONS:

Mix all ingredients except for spray butter and brown sugar in an oven-proof bowl. Spray oatmeal with butter and sprinkle with brown sugar. Bake at 350 degrees for 30 minutes.

Serving: 1
Prep Time: 3 minutes
Cook Time: 30 minutes

This might be a good first step for those a little leery of trying new things in their oatmeal. This is good olf-fashioned oatmeal.

NUTRITION:

Calories 241 | Fat 4.5g | Sodium 140.57mg | Carbs 42.4g | Fiber 5.78g
Sugars 10.75g | Protein 8.84g

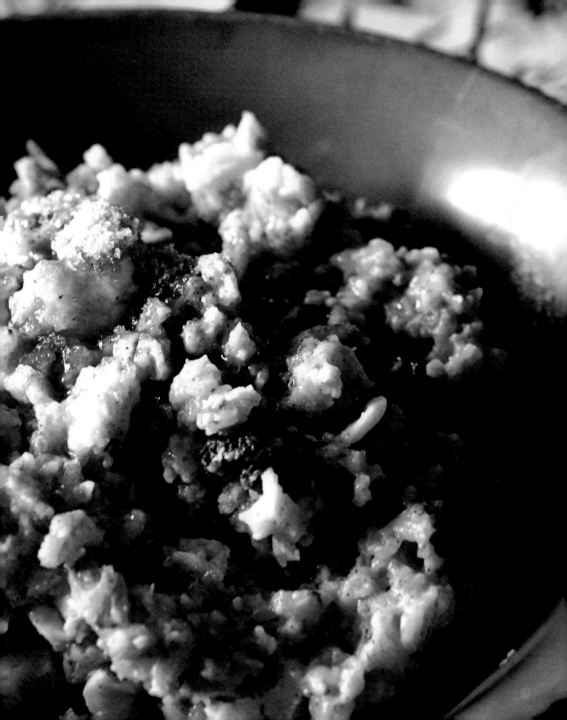

GOLDEN FIG BAKED OATMEAL

INGREDIENTS:

2 Golden Figs, chopped

½ cup old-fashioned oats

½ tsp vanilla

1 Tbsp Bob's creamy hot brown
rice cereal

¼ tsp baking powder

1 cup water

2 Tbsp Torani sugar-free Brown
Sugar and Cinnamon syrup

5 tsp nonfat cottage cheese

DIRECTIONS:

Mix all ingredients except for cottage cheese in an oven-proof bowl. Add dollops of cottage cheese throughout oatmeal. Bake at 350 degrees for 30 to 35 minutes or until oatmeal starts to bubble and pull from edges.

Serving: 1

Prep Time: 3 minutes

Cook Time: 30 minutes

This is one of my all-time favorites. Prior to trying them in baked oatmeal, I had never tried a real fig. I'd had them in Fig Newtons growing up, but that was about the extent of it. Now having tried both dark and light figs, Golden Figs are by far my favorites. This combination is an all-star!

NUTRITION:

Calories 275 | Fat 3.25g | Sodium 76.13mg | Carbs 53.38g | Fiber 7.34g
Sugars 14.96g | Protein 9.12g

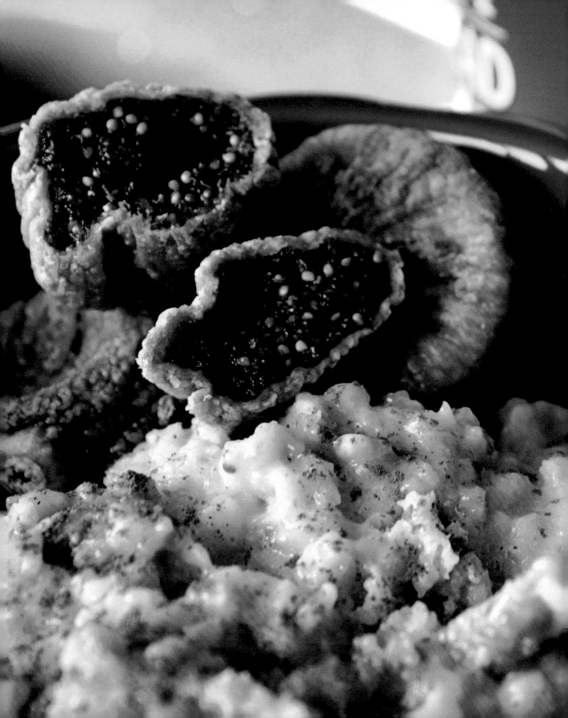

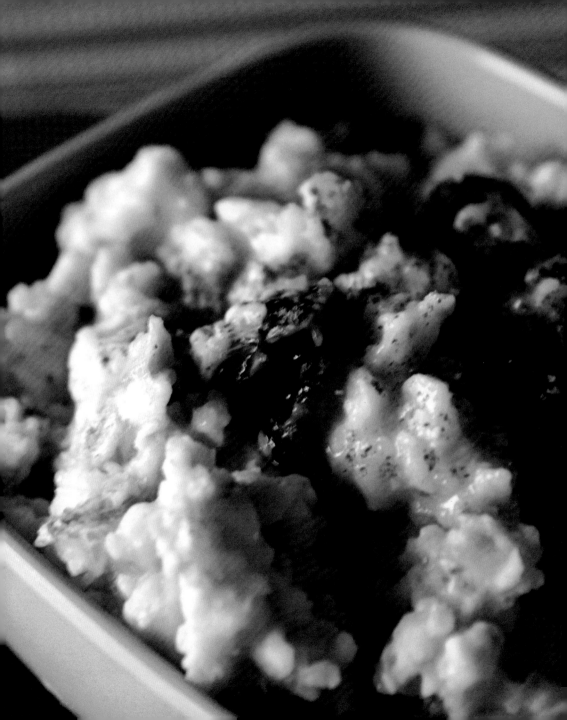

HEARTY HOMEMADE BAKED OATMEAL

INGREDIENTS:

⅓ cup old-fashioned oats

1 cup water

¼ tsp maple extract or mapleine

dash salt

dash cinnamon

Stevia, to taste

2 Tbsp non-fat cottage cheese

1 Tbsp chopped walnuts

1 Tbsp chopped dates

1 Tbsp dried cranberries
   (preferably unsweetened)

1 Tbsp golden raisins

¾ scoop low-carb vanilla
   protein powder

½ tsp baking powder

½ tsp vanilla

DIRECTIONS:

Mix in an oven-proof bowl. Stir well. Bake at 350 degrees for 30 minutes, or until thick.

Serving: 1
Prep Time: 5 minutes
Cook Time: 30 minutes

Every fall I begin craving heartier breakfasts. I'm making my workouts count so that I can enjoy a filling breakfast. On fall mornings I have my baked oatmeal (duh) but as an all-in-one—meaning protein included this time.

NUTRITION:

Calories 376 | Fat 11.37g | Sodium 222.5mg | Carbs 43g | Fiber 4.85g
Sugars 15.87g | Protein 27.83g

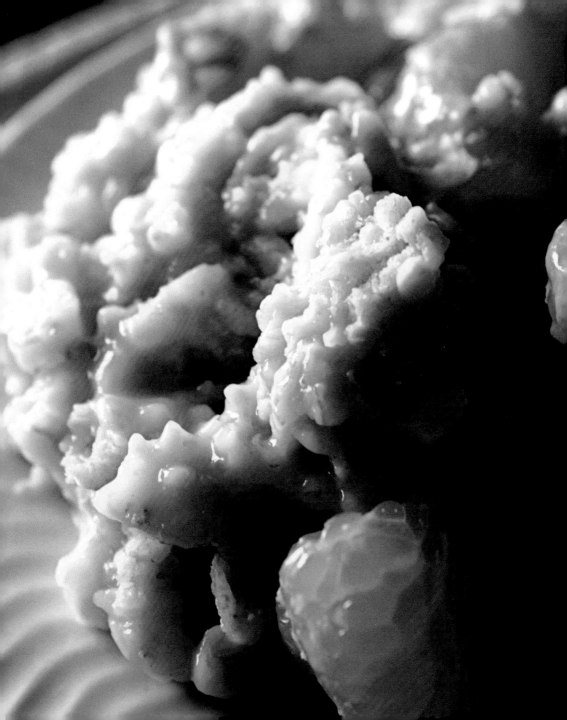

ORANGE COCONUT BAKED OATMEAL

INGREDIENTS:

½ cup old-fashioned oats

¼ tsp baking powder

¼ cup orange juice

¼ cup mandarin oranges

½ tsp imitation coconut flavoring
  (found in baking aisle)

½ tsp vanilla

sugar substitute, to taste

1 cup water

5 tsp nonfat cottage cheese

DIRECTIONS:

Mix in an oven-proof bowl
and bake at 350 degrees for
30 minutes.

Serving: 1
Prep Time: 3 minutes
Cook Time: 30 minutes

Who said you can't try citrus in your oatmeal?

NUTRITION:

Calories 232 | Fat 3.25g | Sodium 79.88mg | Carbs 44.04g | Fiber 4.5g
Sugars 16.12g | Protein 8.7g

JUICY BERRY BAKED OATMEAL

INGREDIENTS:

½ cup old-fashioned oats

1 cup water

2 egg whites

¼ tsp baking powder

2 Tbsp sugar-free Torani
   Raspberry syrup

¼ cup blueberries

4 large strawberries, sliced

sugar substitute, to taste

brown sugar, to taste

DIRECTIONS:

Combine all ingredients except brown sugar in an oven-proof bowl. Bake at 350 degrees for 30 minutes. Remove. Turn oven to broil. Sprinkle small amount of brown sugar on top and broil for an additional 2 to 3 minutes. Remove and enjoy!

Serving: 1
Prep Time: 3 minutes
Cook Time: 30 minutes

This combination is absolutely delicious. It really is so good. The Torani syrup provides a nice subtle berry flavor. The fresh strawberries and blueberries give it lots of juice!

NUTRITION:

Calories 244 | Fat 3g | Sodium 98.25mg | Carbs 43.63g | Fiber 8g
Sugars 13.13g | Protein 10.88g

PEACH COBBLER BAKED OATMEAL

INGREDIENTS:

½ cup old-fashioned oats

¼ tsp baking powder

1 cup water

2 Tbsp sugar-free Torani
Cinnamon Brown Sugar syrup
or Peach syrup

sugar substitute, to taste

2 walnut halves, chopped

½ peach, chopped

DIRECTIONS:

Mix in an oven-proof bowl
and bake at 350 degrees for
30 minutes.

Serving: 1

Prep Time: 5 minutes

Cook Time: 30 minutes

This is so good as is, but if you want to add more texture to it, try adding a small amount of granola and brown sugar at the end. After baking, sprinkle granola and brown sugar on top and broil for a few minutes. It will create a yummy crust! Just be sure to account for the ingredients when calculating nutritional information!

NUTRITION *(without granola and brown sugar)*:
Calories 218 | Fat 6.2g | Sodium 55.1mg | Carbs 32.93g | Fiber 5.34g
Sugars 5.89g | Protein 9.51g

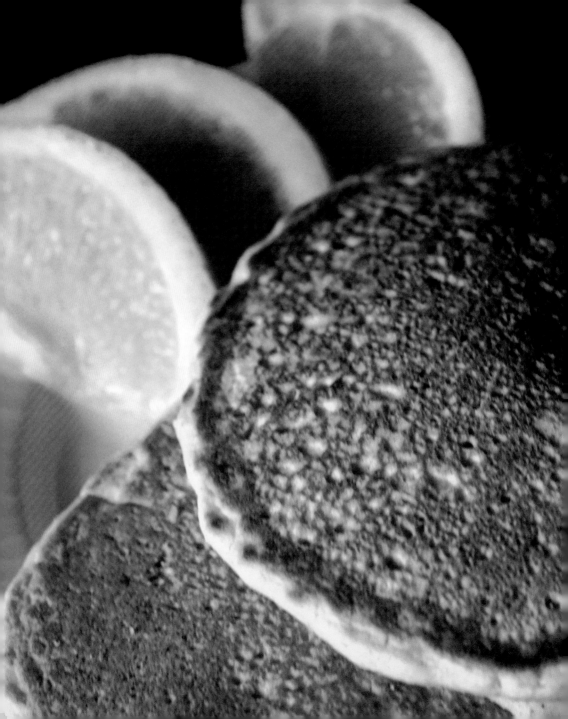

ORANGE OAT PANCAKES

INGREDIENTS:

1 ¼ cups ground oat flour

2 tsp baking powder

1 egg or egg substitute

¾ cup almond milk

¼ cup orange juice

½ tsp salt (optional)

dash orange zest or freshly grated orange peel

dash cinnamon

1 tablespoon sugar substitute (Stevia, Xylitol, honey, agave)

DIRECTIONS:

Sift together flour and baking powder; set aside. Beat together the egg, milk, OJ, salt and sugar in a bowl. Stir in flour until just moistened and stir to incorporate. Coat pan with cooking spray and preheat over medium-high. Pour batter into pan and cook until lightly browned on both sides. Serve.

Serving: 4
Prep Time: 5 minutes
Cook Time: 10 minutes

Just a little addition of orange peel and OJ really makes this. Mmm!

NUTRITION:

Calories 145 | Fat 4.5g | Sodium 413.13mg | Carbs 22.13g | Fiber 3g
Sugars 1.75g | Protein 5.5g

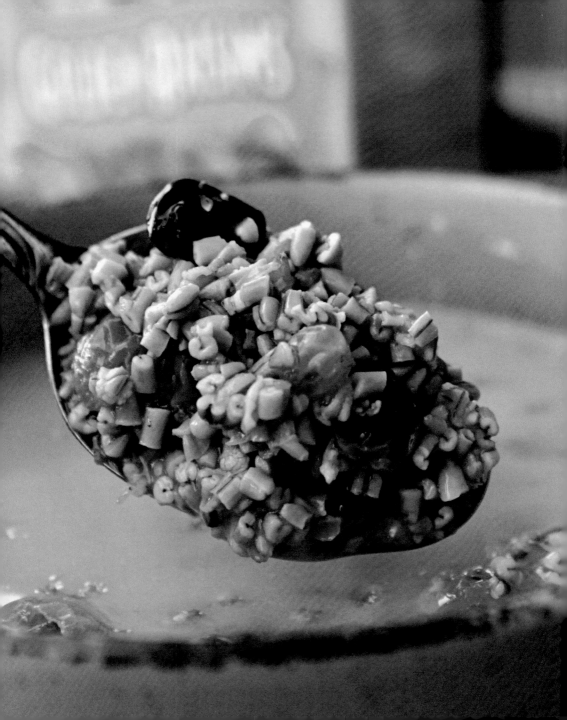

OVERNIGHT NO-COOK CITRUS STEEL CUT OATS

INGREDIENTS:

¾ cup steel cut oats

1 cup almond milk

¾ cup water

2 Tbsp agave nectar or honey

2 Tbsp golden raisins

½ tsp orange zest

dash cinnamon

dash ginger

DIRECTIONS:

Mix in a bowl. Cover in an airtight container and place in fridge overnight until ready to eat in the morning!

Serving: 2

Prep Time: 3 minutes

Soak Time: 7-8 hours

I know there are some of you who like to "cheat" on your oatmeal every now and again. This is another delicious easy night-before breakfast you can grab out of the fridge the morning of with little to no preparation!

NUTRITION:

Calories 336 | Fat 6g | Sodium 90mg | Carbs 60.63g | Fiber 8.75g
Sugars 13.5g | Protein 11.25g

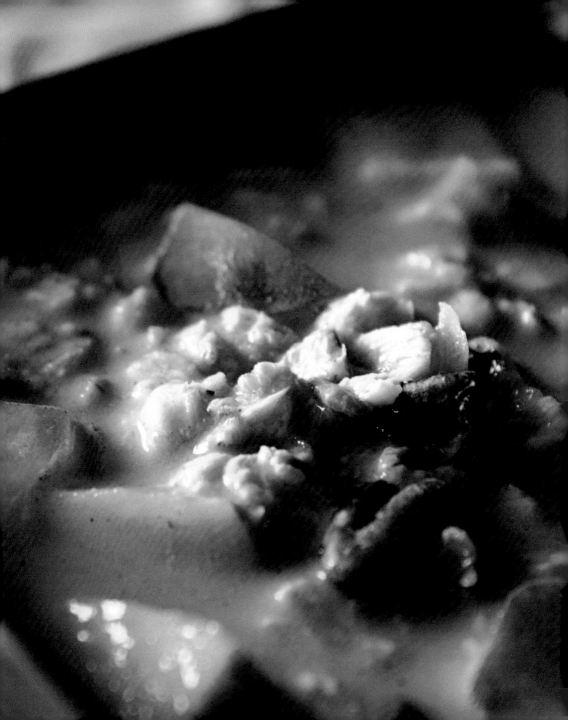

OVERNIGHT NO-COOK PEACH OATMEAL

INGREDIENTS:

½ cup old-fashioned oats

dash cinnamon

dash citrus zest

½ tsp vanilla

1 cup almond milk

1 Tbsp chopped pecans

½ Tbsp agave nectar or honey

½ medium peach, diced

DIRECTIONS:

Combine oats, milk, dash of cinnamon, dash of citrus zest, and tsp vanilla. Soak in an airtight container overnight. The next morning add chopped pecans, sweetener, and diced fresh peaches and serve!

Serving: 1

Prep Time: 3 minutes

Soak Time: 7-8 hours

Not everyone has time to spare in the morning while their oatmeal cooks. This is an easy way to have a great tasting oatmeal with all the work being done the night before.

NUTRITION:

Calories 288 | Fat 11g | Sodium 180mg | Carbs 43g | Fiber 6.75g
Sugars 5.75g | Protein 7.25g

NUTTY OATMEAL BREAKFAST BARS

INGREDIENTS:

2 cups old-fashioned oats

2 medium ripe bananas, mashed

½ cup unsweetened shredded
   coconut

¼ cup chopped walnuts

¼ cup chopped almonds

1 tsp cinnamon

1 tsp apple pie spice

¼ - ⅓ cup unsweetened
   applesauce

2 scoops low-carb nonfat vanilla
   protein powder

DIRECTIONS:

Mix in a medium-sized mixing
bowl. If too thick, add a small
amount of applesauce. Spray a
9" x 9" pan with cooking spray
and pour in batter. Bake at 350
degrees for 25 minutes.

Serving: 9 Bars
Prep Time: 10 minutes
Cook Time: 25 minutes

What I love about oats is they are so much more than just oatmeal. While
oatmeal is and will always be my favorite, I love a good oatmeal bar too.

NUTRITION:

Calories 219 | Fat 10.62g | Sodium 40.06mg | Carbs 22.86g | Fiber 4.48g
Sugars 6.49g | Protein 13.21g

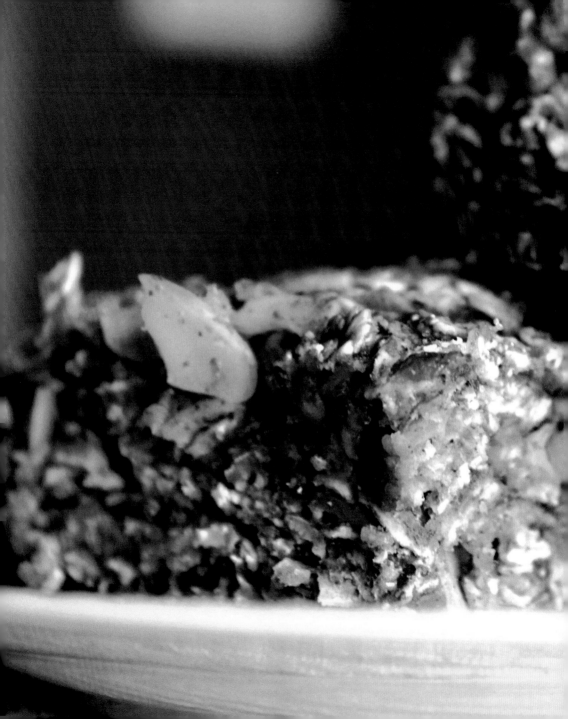

PEANUT BUTTER BAKED OATMEAL W/ CAROB CHIPS

INGREDIENTS:

½ cup old-fashioned oats

2 egg whites

1 cup water

¼ tsp baking powder

sugar substitute, to taste

8 carob chips

1 Tbsp PB2

DIRECTIONS:

Mix in an oven-proof dish and bake at 350 degrees for 30 minutes.

Serving: 1

Prep Time: 10 minutes

Cook Time: 30 minutes

Not quite a Reeses Peanut Butter cup, but it cures the chocolate peanut butter craving.

NUTRITION:

Calories 247 | Fat 8g | Sodium 97mg | Carbs 37g | Fiber 4g | Sugars 8.5g | Protein 9g

RASPBERRY CHEESECAKE BAKED OATMEAL

INGREDIENTS:

½ cup old-fashioned oats

2 Tbsp sugar-free raspberry jam

5 tsp nonfat cottage cheese

4 Cheesecake flavored
  Capella drops

1 Tbsp Torani sugar-free
  Raspberry syrup

1 cup water

¼ tsp baking powder

½ tsp vanilla

sugar substitute

Walden Farms 0-calorie
chocolate sauce

DIRECTIONS:

Mix oats, jam, water, baking powder, Capella drops, Torani syrup, and sugar substitute in oven-proof bowl. Add small dollops of jam and cottage cheese to evenly distribute in oatmeal.

Bake at 350 degrees for 30 to 35 minutes or until oatmeal pulls from sides. Once removed from oven, drizzle sparingly with chocolate sauce.

Serving: 1
Prep Time: 3 minutes
Cook Time: 30 minutes

Not quite Cheesecake Factory, but still a breakfast treat!

NUTRITION:
Calories 185 | Fat 3g | Sodium 74.88mg | Carbs 38.04g | Sugars 1.62g | Protein 7.7g

PEANUT BUTTER BANANA SPLIT BAKED OATMEAL

INGREDIENTS:

½ cup old-fashioned oats

1 cup water

2 egg whites

¼ tsp baking powder

½ banana, sliced

4 medium strawberries, sliced

1 Tbsp PB2 powder

5 Banana Split flavored
  Capella drops

sugar substitute, to taste

DIRECTIONS:

Mix in an oven-proof bowl. Bake at 350 degrees for 30 minutes.

Serving: 1
Prep Time: 3 minutes
Cook Time: 30 minutes

Sometimes I miss being oblivious to fats and calories. I could put away the biggest banana split you'd ever seen. This is a simple recipe incorporating some of my favorite flavors from banana splits past.

NUTRITION *(without granola and brown sugar)*:
Calories 249 | Fat 4.5g | Sodium 97mg | Carbs 44.25g | Fiber 6.13g
Sugars 12.54g | Protein 10.79g

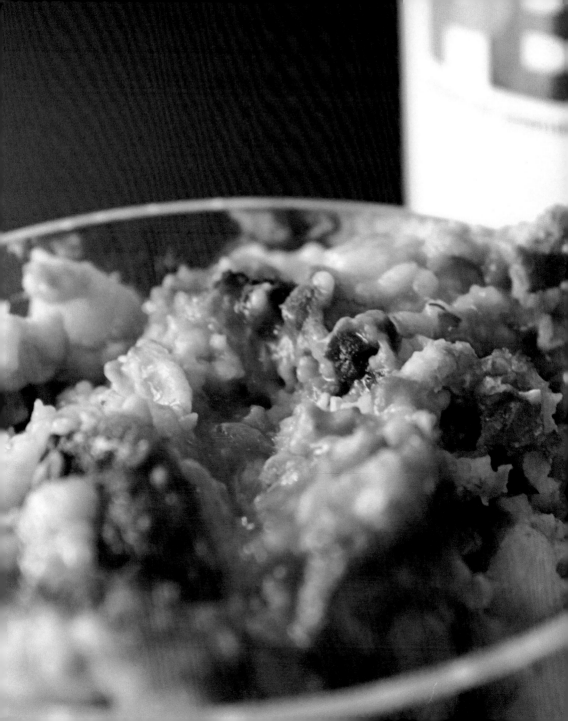

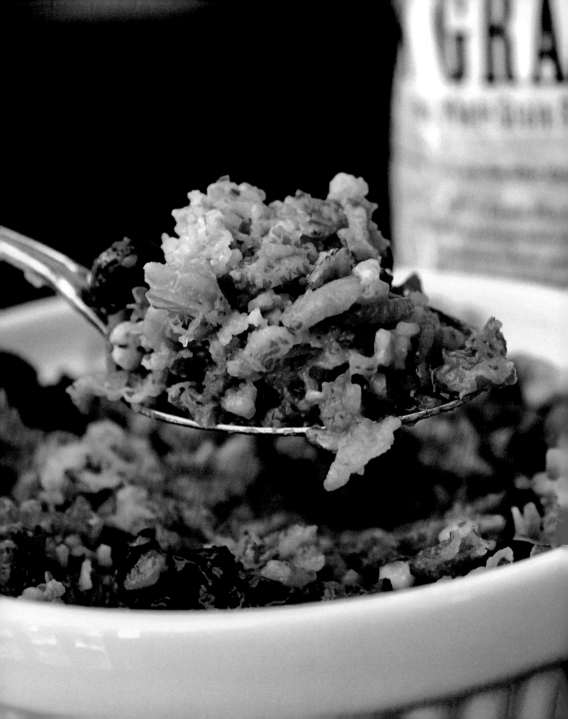

6-GRAIN BLUEBERRY BAKED OATMEAL

INGREDIENTS:

½ cup dry 6-grain oats

5 tsp nonfat cottage cheese

¼ tsp baking powder

1 cup water

¼ cup fresh blueberries

2 Tbsp Torani sugar-free Brown
  Sugar and Cinnamon syrup

½ tsp vanilla

sugar substitute, to taste

DIRECTIONS:

Mix in an oven-proof bowl. Bake at 350 degrees for 30 minutes.

Serving: 1
Prep Time: 3 minutes
Cook Time: 30 minutes

Most health-food stores have a bulk section which is where I found 6-grain oats for this recipe. They are much denser than regular oatmeal. Be sure to allow them to bake up to an additional ten minutes if necessary.

APPROXIMATE NUTRITION:

Calories 232 | Fat 1.7g | Sodium 0mg | Carbs 48.5g | Fiber 1.75g
Sugars 2.5g | Protein 7.05g

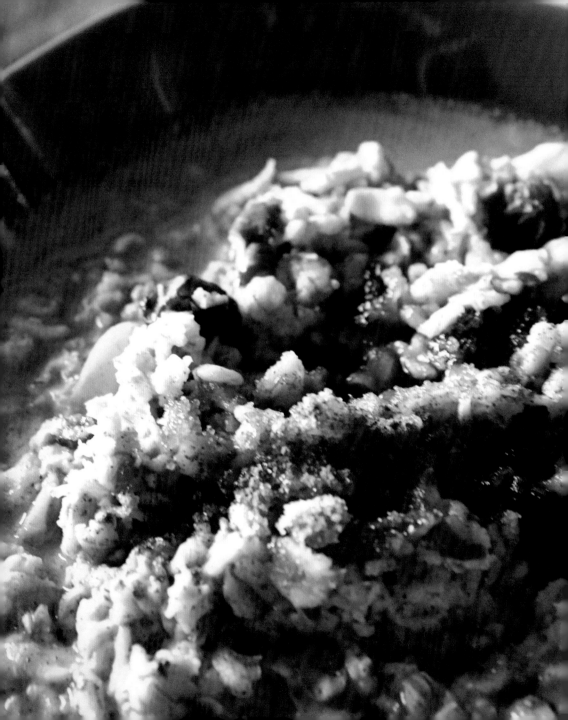

SOAKED OATS

INGREDIENTS:

1 cup old-fashioned oats

1-2 Tbsp lemon juice

1 cup almond milk

pinch salt

2 tsp cinnamon

¼ cup pecans or other nuts

¼ cup raisins

Haven't you ever wondered what oats would taste like if you just let them soak forever? I did. And I tried it. Not bad!

DIRECTIONS:

Add oats to a small bowl. Add enough water to cover; add lemon juice. Soak overnight. In the morning, drain oats and rinse them well. Add milk to a pot and bring to a boil over medium-high heat. Reduce heat. Add remaining ingredients and stir well. Continue to stir until desired thickness. Serve with yogurt and sweetener of your choice.

Serving: 2

Prep Time: 3 minutes

Soak Time: 7-8 hours

NUTRITION:

Calories 360 | Fat 15.2g | Sodium 81.72mg | Carbs 50.91g | Fiber 7.27g
Sugars 21.09g | Protein 7.54g

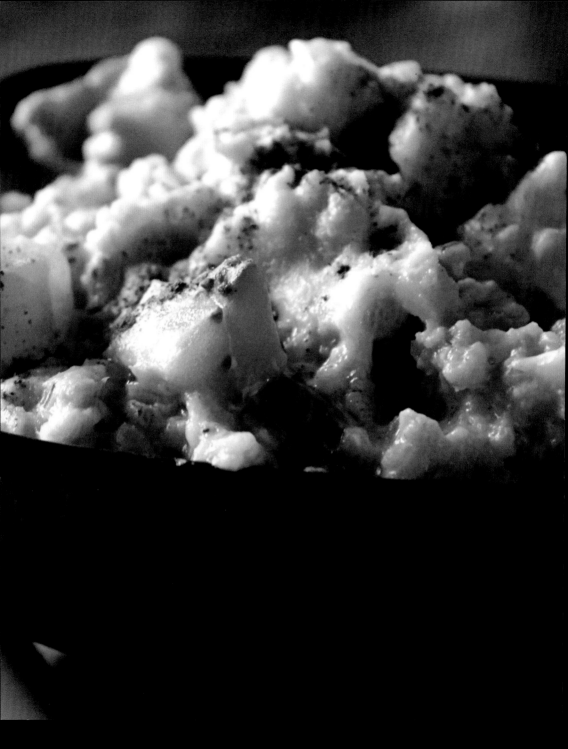

STRAWBERRIES AND CREAM BAKED OATMEAL

INGREDIENTS:

½ cup old-fashioned oats

1 cup water

2 egg whites

¼ tsp baking powder

½ tsp vanilla

pinch salt

sugar substitute, to taste

4-5 strawberries, sliced

Cinnamon, to taste

1-2 Tbsp fat-free half and half

pinch brown sugar

DIRECTIONS:

Mix all but last two ingredients in an oven-proof bowl. Bake at 350 degrees for 30 minutes. Once done, remove from oven, sprinkle with a little brown sugar and broil for 2-3 minutes longer. Top with fat-free half and half.

Serving: 1
Prep Time: 5 minutes
Cook Time: 30 minutes

One of my favorite desserts is strawberry shortcake. I also love fresh sliced strawberries soaked in sweet cream. I made a healthier version and called it breakfast. Enjoy!

NUTRITION:

Calories 242 | Fat 3g | Sodium 142.33mg | Carbs 39.94g | Fiber 5.5g
Sugars 6.5g | Protein 14.5g

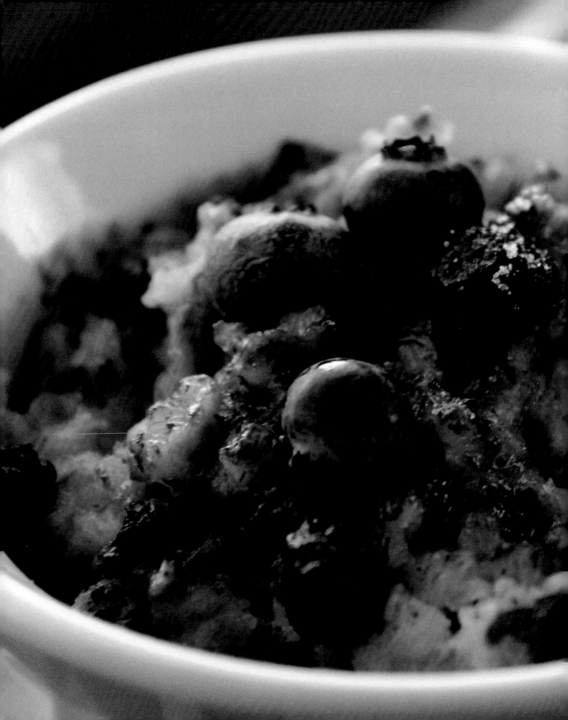

THE 1ST BAKED BLUEBERRY OATMEAL (THE ORIGINAL)

INGREDIENTS:

½ cup old-fashioned oats

1 cup of water

2 egg whites

¼ tsp baking powder

sugar substitute, to taste

10-12 fresh blueberries

cinnamon, to taste

pinch raw sugar

DIRECTIONS:

Mix all but last ingredient in an oven-proof bowl and bake at 350 degrees for 30 minutes. Remove oatmeal from oven and sprinkle with raw sugar. Turn oven to broil and broil for 2-3 minutes until sugar starts to caramelize.

Serving: 1
Prep Time: 3 minutes
Cook Time: 30 minutes

Here's what started it all. My first baked oatmeal. Who knew it would lead to more than two month's worth of baked oatmeal recipes?

NUTRITION:

Calories 169 | Fat 3g | Sodium 0mg | Carbs 29.24g | Fiber 4.15g
Sugars 1g | Protein 5.01g

BLUEBERRY CHEESECAKE BAKED OATMEAL

INGREDIENTS:

½ cup old-fashioned oats

1 cup water

¼ tsp baking powder

1 tsp vanilla

¼ cup fresh blueberries

2 Tbsp Torani sugar-free
    Raspberry or Caramel syrup

sugar substitute, to taste

2 egg whites

5 tsp fat-free cream cheese

DIRECTIONS:

Mix all but last ingredient in an oven-proof bowl. Cut cream cheese in. Bake at 350 degrees for 30 minutes.

Serving: 1
Prep Time: 3 minutes
Cook Time: 30 minutes

Take advantage of fresh blueberries when they are in season when you make this. Nothing compares.

NUTRITION:

Calories 263 | Fat 4.17g | Sodium 548.99mg | Carbs 36.58g | Fiber 5.75g
Sugars 4.08g | Protein 20.5g

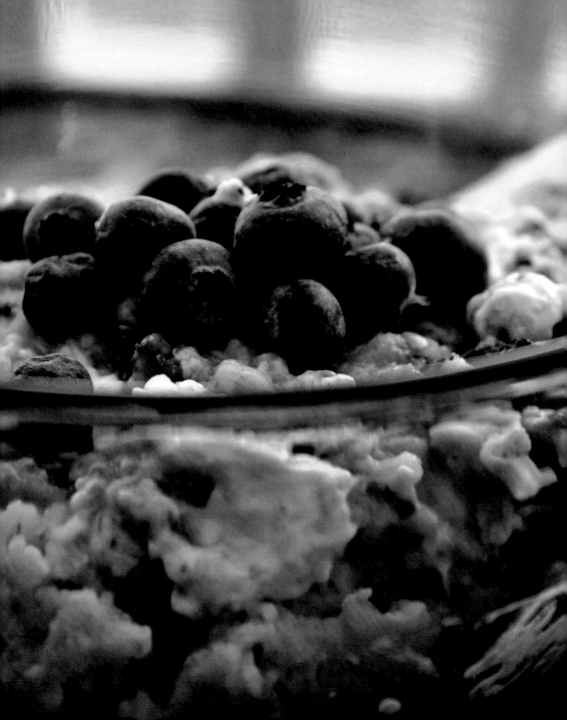

BLUEBERRY LATTE BAKED OATMEAL

INGREDIENTS:

⅓ cup old-fashioned oats

½ scoop low-carb vanilla protein powder

2 Tbsp crushed Fiber One cereal

¾ cup water

1 Tbsp sugar-free Torani Coffee syrup

10 fresh or frozen blueberries

5 tsp nonfat cottage cheese

2 egg whites

¼ tsp baking powder

sugar substitute, to taste

DIRECTIONS:

Combine in an oven-proof bowl. Bake at 350 degrees for 30 minutes.

Serving: 1
Prep Time: 3 minutes
Cook Time: 30 minutes

Sounds like an odd combination, I know, but it's actually really good. Also good with fresh raspberries.

NUTRITION:

Calories 259 | Fat 4.25g | Sodium 214.58mg | Carbs 38.96g | Fiber 8.93g
Sugars 3.87g | Protein 21.16g

CHERRY CRANBERRY TART BAKED OATMEAL

INGREDIENTS:

½ cup old-fashioned oats

1 cup water

¼ cup pitted and halved cherries
   (fresh or frozen)

2 Tbsp sweetened dried
   cranberries

¼ tsp lemon juice

½ tsp vanilla

¼ tsp baking powder

sugar substitute, to taste

Tart and more tart. Yum.

DIRECTIONS:

Combine in an oven-proof bowl. Bake at 350 degrees for 30 minutes.

Serving: 1
Prep Time: 5 minutes
Cook Time: 30 minutes

NUTRITION:

Calories 227 | Fat 3.08g | Sodium 0mg | Carbs 46.33g | Fiber 5.48g
Sugars 17.25g | Protein 5.38g

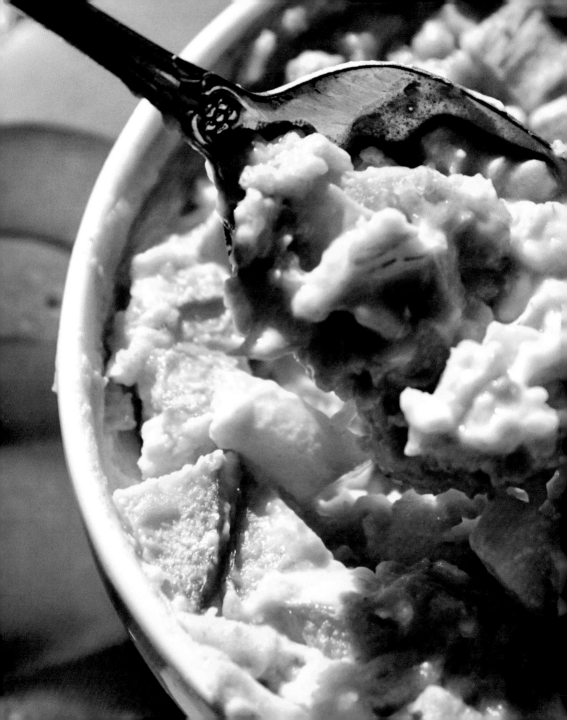

CHEESY PEACH-ON-PEACH BAKED OATMEAL

INGREDIENTS:

½ cup old-fashioned oats

½ peach, thinly sliced

2 egg whites

¼ tsp baking powder

dash salt

3 Tbsp sugar-free Torani
   Peach syrup

3 Tbsp nonfat cottage cheese

1 cup water

sugar substitute, to taste

DIRECTIONS:

Mix in an oven-proof bowl. Bake at 350 degrees for 30 minutes.

Serving: 1
Prep Time: 5 minutes
Cook Time: 30 minutes

This was the first baked oatmeal recipe I tried with cottage cheese. Since trying it with, I've never gone a day without. I like it that much. It makes the oatmeal "meatier," if that even makes sense.

NUTRITION:

Calories 211 | Fat 3g | Sodium 185mg | Carbs 34.13g | Fiber 5g
Sugars 6.88g | Protein 13.63g

CINNAMON CHOCOLATE CHIP BAKED OATMEAL

INGREDIENTS:

½ cup old-fashioned oats

1 cup water

¼ tsp baking powder

2 Tbsp Torani sugar-free Chocolate Chip Cookie Dough syrup

2 Tbsp Torani sugar-free White Chocolate syrup

2 egg whites

5 tsp nonfat cottage cheese

24 carob chips

1 Tbsp chopped walnuts

½ tsp vanilla

dash cinnamon

sugar substitute, to taste

DIRECTIONS:

Mix in an oven-proof bowl. Bake at 350 degrees for 30 minutes.

Serving: 1
Prep Time: 5 minutes
Cook Time: 30 minutes

My dad introduced me to the Doubletree Hotel's Cinnamon Chocolate Chip cookies several years ago. Ever since then I stay at their hotels whenever I can, and I've even ordered a couple of tins for him at Christmas. Something about the cinnamon and chocolate combination reminds me of my dad. I had that same reminiscent feeling when I made this oatmeal. This one is for Dad.

NUTRITION:

Calories 311 | Fat 12.16g | Sodium 174.83mg | Carbs 37.71g | Fiber 4.67g
Sugars 8.79g | Protein 14.2g

CREAMY PUMPKIN CRANBERRY BAKED OATMEAL

INGREDIENTS:

½ cup old-fashioned oats

1 cup water

3 Tbsp cranberries

¼ tsp baking powder

¼ cup pumpkin puree

3 Tbsp nonfat cottage cheese

¼ tsp cinnamon

¼ tsp ground nutmeg

¼ tsp vanilla

¼ tsp ginger powder

sugar substitute, to taste

DIRECTIONS:

Before preparing oatmeal, boil about a quart of water and cook cranberries in boiling water until they "pop." Remove from heat. Pour water off and save cranberries in a sealed container for future use.

Combine ingredients above in an oven-proof bowl. Bake in a preheated 350-degree oven for 30 minutes.

Serving: 1
Prep Time: 15 minutes
Cook Time: 30 minutes

Two Fall favorites – pumpkin and cranberries – together.

NUTRITION:

Calories 229 | Fat 3.46g | Sodium 163.83mg | Carbs 39.35g | Fiber 8.18g
Sugars 7.6g | Protein 11.28g

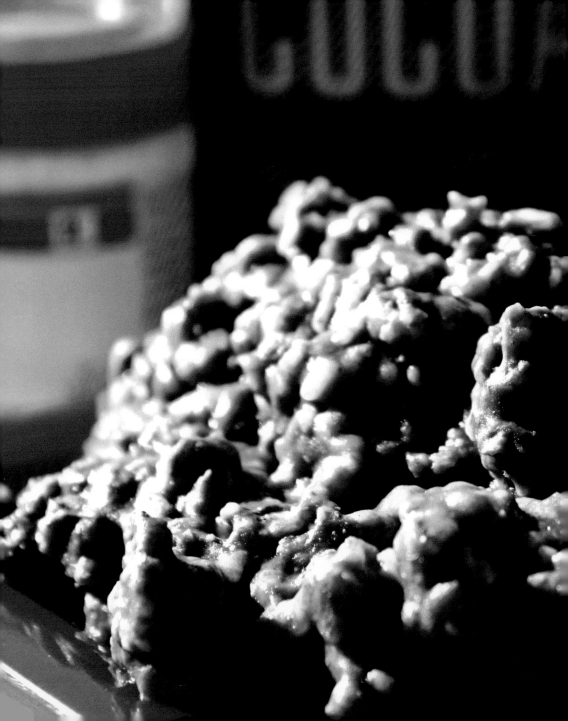

CREAMY CHOCOLATE PUMPKIN BAKED OATMEAL

INGREDIENTS:

½ cup old-fashioned oats

1 cup water

3 Tbsp pumpkin puree

3 Tbsp nonfat cottage cheese

1 Tbsp cocoa powder

¼ tsp baking powder

dash salt

⅛ tsp nutmeg

⅛ tsp cloves

⅛ tsp cinnamon

sugar substitute, to taste

DIRECTIONS:

Combine in an oven-proof bowl. Bake at 350 degrees for 30 minutes.

Serving: 1
Prep Time: 3 minutes
Cook Time: 30 minutes

This reminds me of the fat chocolate pumpkin cookies I make every year around Thanksgiving – only this is healthier.

NUTRITION:

Calories 213 | Fat 3.85g | Sodium 152.59mg | Carbs 36.07g | Fiber 8.03g
Sugars 4.97g | Protein 11.73g

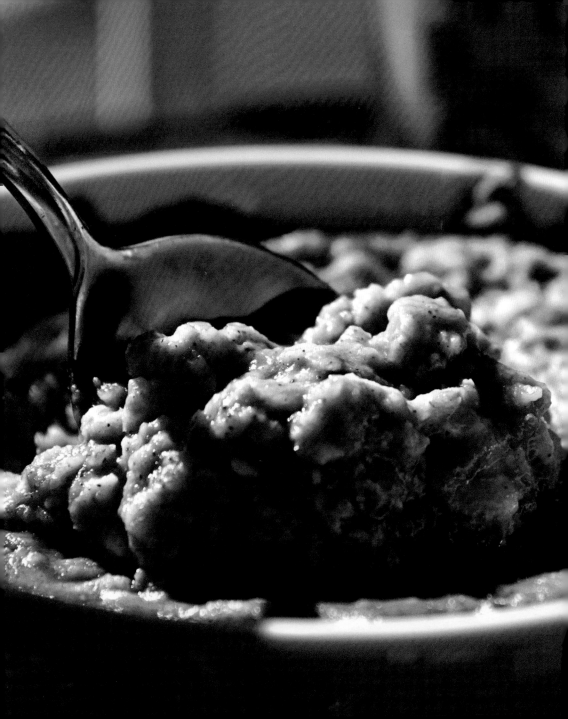

GINGER PUMPKIN BAKED OATMEAL

INGREDIENTS:

½ cup old-fashioned oats

1 cup water

¼ cup pumpkin puree

2 Tbsp nonfat cottage cheese

¼ tsp baking powder

dash salt

¼ tsp cinnamon

½ tsp vanilla

⅛ tsp allspice

1 piece crystallized ginger, crushed

sugar substitute, to taste

DIRECTIONS:

Combine in an oven-proof bowl. Bake at 350 degrees for 30 minutes.

Serving: 1
Prep Time: 3 minutes
Cook Time: 30 minutes

A couple of years ago I started adding crystallized ginger to my pumpkin pies. The two flavors together are delicious. Translates well to baked oatmeal!

NUTRITION:

Calories 213 | Fat 3.22g | Sodium 103.09mg | Carbs 37.51g | Fiber 5.93g
Sugars 9.25g | Protein 9.27g

MAPLE PUMPKIN BAKED OATMEAL

INGREDIENTS:

½ cup old-fashioned oats

1 cup water

¼ cup pumpkin puree

¼ tsp baking powder

1-2 tsp pure maple extract

¼ tsp cinnamon

⅛ tsp nutmeg

3 Tbsp nonfat cottage cheese

sugar substitute, to taste

DIRECTIONS:

Combine in an oven-proof bowl. Bake at 350 degrees for 30 minutes.

Serving: 1
Prep Time: 3 minutes
Cook Time: 30 minutes

I used Mapeline (imitation maple extract) in this recipe, but you could also use a little bit of 100% maple syrup or sugar-free maple syrup. You'll love it!

NUTRITION:

Calories 202 | Fat 3.36g | Sodium 163.79mg | Carbs 34.27g | Fiber 6.56g
Sugars 5.71g | Protein 11.27g

PUMPKIN PIE BAKED OATMEAL

INGREDIENTS:

½ cup old-fashioned oats

¼ cup pumpkin puree

3 Tbsp nonfat cottage cheese

2 Tbsp chopped dates

¼ tsp pumpkin pie spice

½ tsp vanilla

¼ tsp cinnamon

sugar substitute, to taste

1 cup water

¼ tsp baking powder

2 Tbsp sugar-free Torani
   Gingersnap syrup

DIRECTIONS:

Combine in an oven-proof bowl.
Bake at 350 degrees for 30
minutes.

Serving: 1
Prep Time: 3 minutes
Cook Time: 30 minutes

Every year I look forward to fall. I love the bright colors on the trees, I love the cloud cover, I love to decorate my home, I love the abundant smells. I love everything about it. Recently I discovered something new I love about fall: Pumpkin Pie Baked Oatmeal. This is a real treat and it isn't just for fall.

NUTRITION:

Calories 260 | Fat 3.25g 5% | Sodium 178.75mg | Carbs 49.63g | Fiber 8g
Sugars 18.63g | Protein 11.75g

APPLE PEANUT BUTTER BAKED OATMEAL

INGREDIENTS:

⅔ cup quick-cooking oats

3 egg whites

1 cup water

1 ½ Tbsp PB2

⅓ cup apple pie filling or
   apple slices

⅛ tsp baking soda

dash salt

sugar substitute, to taste

DIRECTIONS:

Mix in an oven-proof bowl. Bake at 350 degrees for 30 minutes.

Serving: 1
Prep Time: 5 minutes
Cook Time: 30 minutes

This yummy concoction came from one of my Facebook fans, Sue Ann Bernard. Thanks Sue for this great baked oatmeal recipe!

NUTRITION:

Calories 256 | Fat 4.46g | Sodium 145.5mg | Carbs 40.14g | Fiber 6.84g
Sugars 2.46g | Protein 16.63g

CHOCONANA BAKED OATMEAL

INGREDIENTS:

⅓ cup old-fashioned oats

¾ cup water

5 tsp nonfat cottage cheese

¼ tsp baking powder

½ tsp vanilla

1 tsp dark chocolate baking chips

1 Tbsp sugar-free Torani
  chocolate syrup

½ banana, sliced

sugar substitute, to taste

DIRECTIONS:

Mix everything except for the chocolate chips and cottage cheese in an oven-proof bowl. Once mixed, add dollops of cottage cheese and chips sparingly throughout oatmeal. Bake at 350 degrees for 30 minutes.

Serving: 1
Prep Time: 5 minutes
Cook Time: 30 minutes

One word, "yum!"

NUTRITION:

Calories 307 | Fat 5.5g | Sodium 203.55mg | Carbs 41.02g | Fiber 6g
Sugars 14.62g | Protein 25.87g

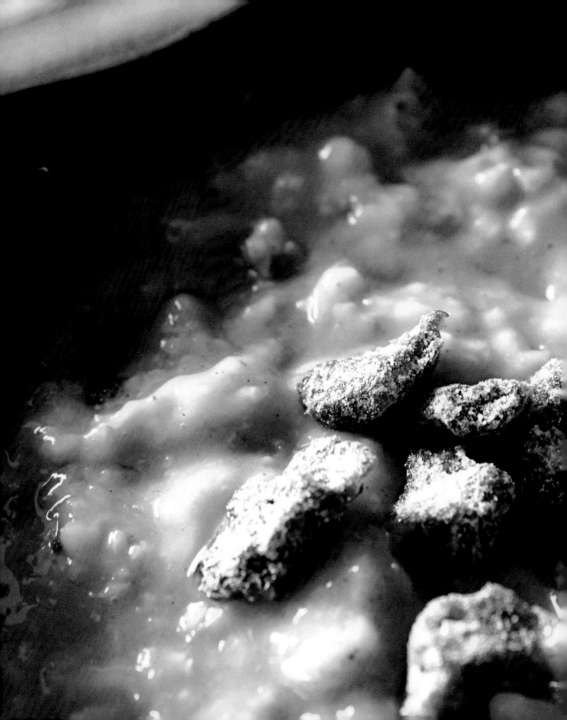

CROCKPOT COMPANY FRUIT OATMEAL

INGREDIENTS:

1 cup old-fashioned oats

½ cup almond milk

4 cups water

1 tsp vanilla

1 Tbsp dried cranberries

1 Tbsp raisins

2 dates, chopped

2 dried apricots, chopped

sugar substitute, to taste

DIRECTIONS:

Coat inside of Crockpot with cooking spray. Mix ingredients inside pot and cover. Cook on low for 7-8 hours.

Drizzle hot oatmeal with additional almond milk and cinnamon.

Serving: 2
Prep Time: 5 minutes
Cook Time: 6-7 hours

You can double or triple this depending on how much you need. Since it has all night to cook through, you can rest assured knowing it will be ready!

NUTRITION:

Calories 305 | Fat 5.25g | Sodium 49.68mg | Carbs 58.72g | Fiber 7.67g
Sugars 16.24g | Protein 8.22g

DRIED PINEAPPLE AND CHERRY BAKED OATMEAL

INGREDIENTS:

½ cup old-fashioned oats

1 cup water

¼ tsp baking powder

3 dried pineapple wedges,
  cut into thin slices

7 dried cherries, cut into pieces

1 Tbsp Torani sugar-free
  Coconut syrup

1 Tbsp Torani sugar-free
  Dark Cherry syrup

1 Tbsp Torani sugar-free
  Cinnamon and Sugar syrup

5 tsp nonfat cottage cheese

½ tsp pure vanilla extract

1 Tbsp crushed Fiber One cereal

sugar substitute, to taste

DIRECTIONS:

Mix all but last two ingredients in oven-proof bowl. Once combined, add dollops of cottage cheese to top and sprinkle with crushed Fiber One. Bake at 350 degrees for 30 minutes.

Serving: 1
Prep Time: 5 minutes
Cook Time: 30 minutes

Christmas Fruit Bars baked oatmeal style. Enjoy!

NUTRITION:

Calories 255 | Fat 3.13g | Sodium 96.67mg | Carbs 53.42g | Fiber 7.14g
Sugars 19.41g | Protein 8.35g

OVERNIGHT MIXED-GRAIN OATMEAL

INGREDIENTS:

¼ cup old-fashioned oats

2 Tbsp brown rice

2 Tbsp barley

¼ cup chopped dried strawberries

¼ cup chopped dried apples

1 tsp vanilla

1 tsp cinnamon

3 cups water

sugar substitute, to taste

DIRECTIONS:

Coat inside of Crockpot with cooking spray. Mix ingredients inside pot and cover. Cook on low for 7-8 hours.

Drizzle hot oatmeal with almond milk and cinnamon, to taste.

Serving: 2
Prep Time: 5 minutes
Cook Time: 6-7 hours

This is another fun recipe to help mix things up. We automatically think we need to switch up the fruit and seasonings. We can also play around by changing the grains – like in this one!

NUTRITION:

Calories 263 | Fat 1.13g | Sodium 26.38mg | Carbs 62.25g | Fiber 8.07g
Sugars 38.77g | Protein 3.33g

MY FAVORITE CROCKPOT OATMEAL

INGREDIENTS:

⅔ cup steel cut oats

5 cups water

⅔ cup barley

½ sliced banana

½ diced apple

3 Tbsp unsweetened organic
    applesauce

1 tsp vanilla

½ tsp cinnamon

2 Tbsp chopped almonds

2 Tbsp dried cranberries

3 Tbsp Torani sugar-free Brown
    Sugar & Cinnamon syrup

dash salt

DIRECTIONS:

Coat inside of Crockpot with cooking spray. Mix ingredients inside pot and cover. Cook on low for 7-8 hours.

Drizzle hot oatmeal with almond milk and cinnamon, to taste.

Serving: 3

Prep Time: 5 minutes

Cook Time: 6-7 hours

This crockpot recipe has a little bit of everything. That's what I love about it.

NUTRITION:

Calories 332 | Fat 5.39g | Sodium 197.46mg | Carbs 63.67g | Fiber 9.55g
Sugars 10.46g | Protein 4.52g

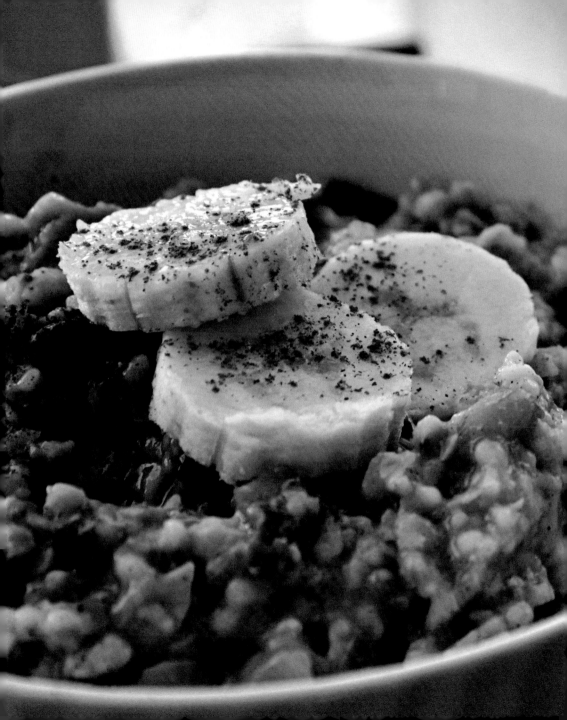

PEACH STRUDEL BAKED OATMEAL

INGREDIENTS:

½ cup old-fashioned oats

1 medium sliced peach

2 Tbsp crushed Fiber One cereal

1 Tbsp raisins

3 Tbsp nonfat cottage cheese

2 Tbsp sugar-free Torani English
   Toffee syrup

2 egg whites

¼ tsp baking powder

1 cup water

dash salt

sugar substitute, to taste

DIRECTIONS:

Mix in an oven-proof bowl. Bake
at 350 degrees for 30 minutes.

Serving: 1

Prep Time: 5 minutes

Cook Time: 30 minutes

This cereal really makes a difference. You'll love it!

NUTRITION:

Calories 275 | Fat 3.25g | Sodium 164.61mg | Carbs 55.54g | Fiber 10.22g
Sugars 20.87g | Protein: 11.71g

RASPBERRY AND CREAM CHEESE BAKED OATMEAL

INGREDIENTS:

½ cup old-fashioned oats

5 tsp fat-free cream cheese

¼ tsp baking powder

½ tsp vanilla

¼ cup fresh or frozen raspberries

1 cup water

2 egg whites

sugar substitute, to taste

DIRECTIONS:

Cut cream cheese in to bowl of oats. Combine with the other ingredients in an oven-proof bowl. Bake at 350 degrees for 30 minutes. Drizzle with almond milk, to taste.

Serving: 1

Prep Time: 3 minutes

Cook Time: 30 minutes

If you like the raspberry taste but not the seeds, use Torani's sugar-free Raspberry flavoring or a raspberry seedless jelly.

NUTRITION:

Calories 211 | Fat 3.33g | Sodium 179.12mg | Carbs 34.58g | Fiber 5.25g
Sugars 5.08g | Protein 12.17g

TART CHERRY AND BLUEBERRY BAKED OATMEAL

INGREDIENTS:

½ cup old-fashioned oats

¼ tsp baking powder

1 cup water

2 Tbsp sugar-free Torani Dark
   Cherry syrup

⅓ cup chopped fresh cherries

¼ cup fresh blueberries

1 Tbsp crushed Fiber One

5 tsp nonfat cottage cheese

sugar substitute, to taste

DIRECTIONS:

Combine in an oven-proof bowl.
Bake at 350 degrees for 30
minutes.

Serving: 1
Prep Time: 5 minutes
Cook Time: 30 minutes

If cherries aren't in season, buy frozen or pie-filling cherries. Just be sure
to rinse them well to remove the heavy syrup before adding them to your
baked oatmeal.

NUTRITION:

Calories 244 | Fat 4.97g | Sodium 89.26mg | Carbs 44.37g | Fiber 9.99g
Sugars 10.08g | Protein 9.7g

CINNAMON COCONUT GRANOLA

INGREDIENTS:

2 cups quick oats

½ cup oat bran

⅓ cup flaked unsweetened coconut

⅓ cup slivered almonds

3 Tbsp light coconut milk

1 Tbsp organic coconut oil

3 Tbsp honey or agave nectar

3 Tbsp barley malt syrup

3 Tbsp golden raisins

1 tsp vanilla

1 tsp cinnamon

DIRECTIONS:

Preheat oven to 350 degrees. Mix oats, oat bran, coconut, and almonds. Lay out flat on cookie sheet. Bake for 8 minutes in oven until golden brown. Allow to cool and then return to the original bowl.

While the oats are toasting, combine milk, oil, syrup, cinnamon, and honey in a small saucepan. Cook over medium heat until boiling. Allow to boil for a couple of minutes before removing. Stir in vanilla. Pour the hot syrup mixture over oat mixture until completely coated. Spread out on pan again and bake for another 8 minutes. Once removed from the oven, allow to cool and then toss in raisins.

Serving: 6   Prep Time: 10 minutes   Cook Time: 15-20 minutes

NUTRITION:

Calories: 301 | Fat: 11.5g | Sodium: 0mg | Carbs: 47.01g | Fiber: 6.05g
Sugars: 16.42g | Protein: 7.79g

TROPICAL BAKED OATMEAL

INGREDIENTS:

½ cup old-fashioned oats

1 cup water

¼ tsp baking powder

⅓ banana, sliced

5 tsp nonfat cottage cheese

½ Tbsp flaked unsweetened
   coconut

½ tsp imitation coconut flavoring

3 Tbsp Torani sugar-free
   Mango syrup

sugar substitute, to taste

DIRECTIONS:

Combine in an oven-safe bowl and
at 350 degrees for 30 minutes.

Serving: 1

Prep Time: 3 minutes

Cook Time: 30 minutes

My vacation of choice is anywhere tropical. Oatmeal doesn't replace a
vacation, but takes me there even if only momentarily! You could also add
some fresh mango and papaya if in season!

NUTRITION:

Calories 219 | Fat 4.5g | Sodium 74.88mg | Carbs 38.45g | Fiber 5.83g
Sugars 8.62g | Protein 8.04g

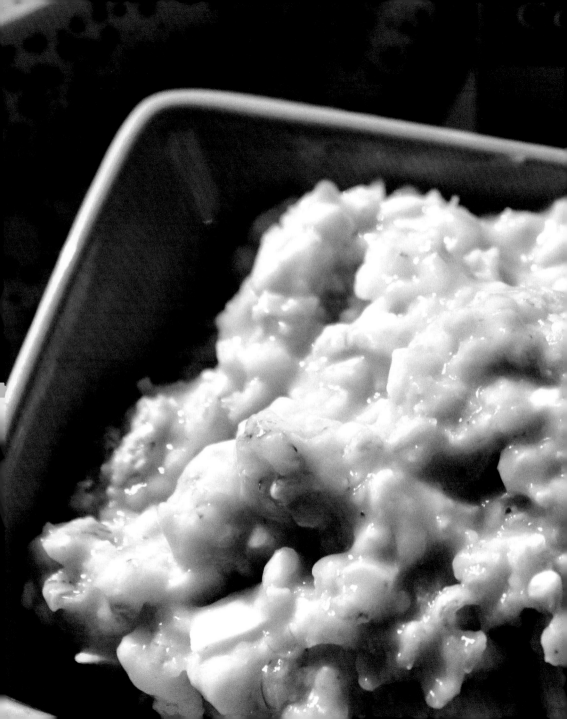

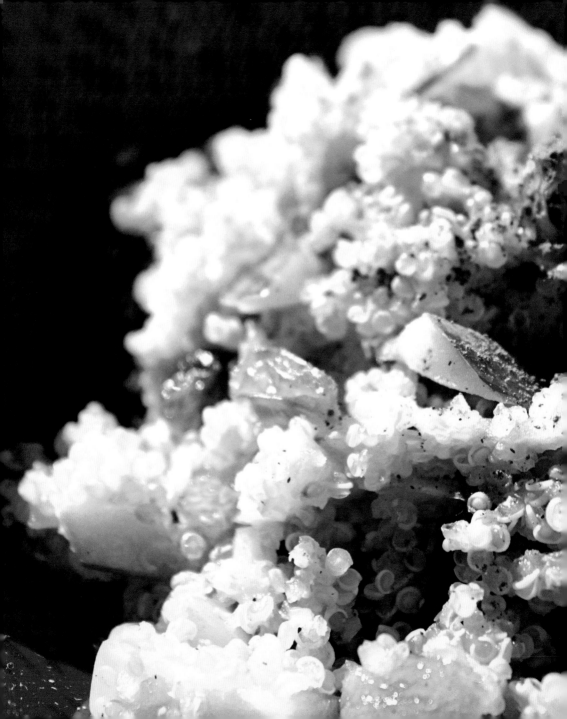

APPLE PIE QUINOA

INGREDIENTS:

½ cup uncooked quinoa

1 cup water

½ Tbsp Smart Balance
  50/50 butter

½ medium apple, diced

2 Tbsp slivered almonds

2 Tbsp golden raisins

1 Tbsp agave nectar

dash cinnamon or apple pie spice

DIRECTIONS:

Bring the quinoa and water to a boil in a saucepan over high heat. Reduce heat to medium-low, cover, and simmer until the quinoa is tender and the water has been absorbed, about 15 to 20 minutes. Melt the butter in a large skillet over medium heat. Add the apple, raisins, and almonds. Drizzle with agave nectar. Cook over medium-low heat for 2 to 3 minutes or until apples start to soften up. Stir the apple mixture into cooked quinoa. Sprinkle with cinnamon or apple pie spice and serve!

Serving: 1

Prep Time: 5 minutes

Cook Time: 20-25 minutes

America's favorite pie with a GREAT oat alternative.

NUTRITION:

Calories 307 | Fat 8.75g | Sodium 24.75mg | Carbs 50.25g | Fiber 5.75g
Sugars 14.5g | Protein 7.63g

CREAMY RICE HOT PROTEIN CEREAL

INGREDIENTS:

¼ cup Creamy Rice Hot Cereal

1 scoop BSN Lean Dessert Fresh Cinnamon Roll protein powder (or favorite)

1 Tbsp flax seed

water, for boiling

almond milk, to taste (optional)

DIRECTIONS:

Follow package directions for hot cereal. When nearly done, mix in flax seed and protein powder. Add small amount of water or almond milk if too thick. Enjoy!

Serving: 1
Prep Time: 2 minutes
Cook Time: 1-10 minutes

Before I tried oatmeal, I ate Bob's Creamy Rice Hot Cereal and a lot of it! This was meal number one for nearly a full year. I never got tired of it. If you haven't tried rice cereal, it's very similar to porridge. It has a smooth, creamy consistency. Like with the oatmeal shake, I loved this with BSN Lean Dessert's Fresh Cinnamon Roll. Breakfast just made my morning. You can try it with whatever your favorite is though.

NUTRITION:

Calories: 330 | Fat: 7.5g | Sodium: 107.5 | Carbs: 42.5g | Fiber: 6g
Sugars: 3g | Protein: 25g

DRY CINNAMON OATMEAL SNACK

INGREDIENTS:

1 cup old-fashioned oats

¼ tsp cinnamon

sugar substitute, to taste

I debated whether I should even include this recipe because there's really nothing to it. Then I realized how many times this little snack has saved my butt—literally—in times of temptation. My posing coach, and initial diet trainer, Sandy Hancock, turned me on to this little mix. I remember when I read it on the diet, I asked, "Do I really eat it dry?" I was shocked and skeptical. Little did I know I'd start taking it with me everywhere—even on long vacations.

DIRECTIONS:

Mix everything in a Ziploc baggie and throw in a plastic spoon. Instant snack.

Lately I've also been adding a small amount of PB2 for a peanut butter flavor. Other times I'll sprinkle in some flavored protein powder—whatever sounds good. Regardless, it's a healthy snack for when you're on the go.

Serving: 2

Prep Time: 2 minutes

NUTRITION:

Calories: 150 | Fat: 3gSugars: 3gSodium: 0mg | Carbs: 27g | Fiber: 4g
Sugars: 1g | Protein: 5g

FRUITY ALMOND MUESLI

INGREDIENTS:

1 cup old-fashioned oats

½ cup shredded wheat

¼ cup unsweetened dried
   cranberries

¼ cup chopped dried apricots

¼ cup dried blueberries

¼ cup slivered almonds

2 Tbsp ground flaxseed

2 Tbsp toasted wheat germ

1 tsp cinnamon

1 Tbsp Stevia granular

DIRECTIONS:

Combine in a bowl. Keep in
an airtight container for up to
a month.

Serving: 4

Prep Time: 3 minutes

With so many healthy ingredients loaded in one snack, you can't go wrong.
Eat this alone or add Greek Yogurt or Almond Milk.

NUTRITION:

Calories: 227 | Fat: 6.87g | Sodium: 1mg | Carbs: 35.41g | Sugars: 9.38g | Protein: 6.56g

OATMEAL PROTEIN SHAKE

INGREDIENTS:

½ cup old-fashioned oats

1 scoop BSN Lean Dessert Fresh
   Cinnamon Roll protein powder

8 oz water

DIRECTIONS:

Add all ingredients to a shaker cup and shake vigorously. Eat right away or allow oatmeal to soak. Either way, have a spoon handy so you can eat the oatmeal first if desired, or just drink it straight out of the cup!

Serving: 1
Prep Time: 2 minutes

This is another balanced snack for on the go. I took this with me countless times to the pool while my son had swim lessons. It's a quick, easy treat that I've enjoyed and thought you might too. For this recipe I'm suggesting BSN Lean Dessert's Fresh Cinnamon Roll flavored protein powder because that was my favorite at the time—especially when combined with oatmeal. However, anything will work. Find what you like!

NUTRITION:

Calories: 280 | Fat: 6g | Sodium 100mg | Carbs: 34g | Fiber: 5g
Sugars: 4g | Protein: 25g

QUINOA FOR BREAKFAST

INGREDIENTS:

⅓ cup quinoa

¼ tsp ground cinnamon

1 cup almond milk

⅓ cup water (if needed)

1 Tbsp brown sugar/
   Splenda blend

1 tsp vanilla

pinch salt

I bought a huge bag of quinoa at Costco a couple of months ago. I wasn't rotating through it fast enough, so that's when I started getting creative for breakfast.

DIRECTIONS:

Heat a saucepan with milk over medium heat and add quinoa. Season with cinnamon and cook for 3 minutes or until toasted. Add remaining ingredients. Bring to a boil, then cook over low heat until the porridge is thick and grains are tender, about 25 minutes. If quinoa becomes dry, add more water a little bit at a time. Stir constantly, especially at the end when it has a tendency to burn.

Serving: 2
Prep Time: 3 minutes
Cook Time: 25 minutes

NUTRITION:

Calories: 173 | Fat: 3g | Sodium: 219mg | Carbs: 31.3g | Fiber: 3g | Protein: 4.3g

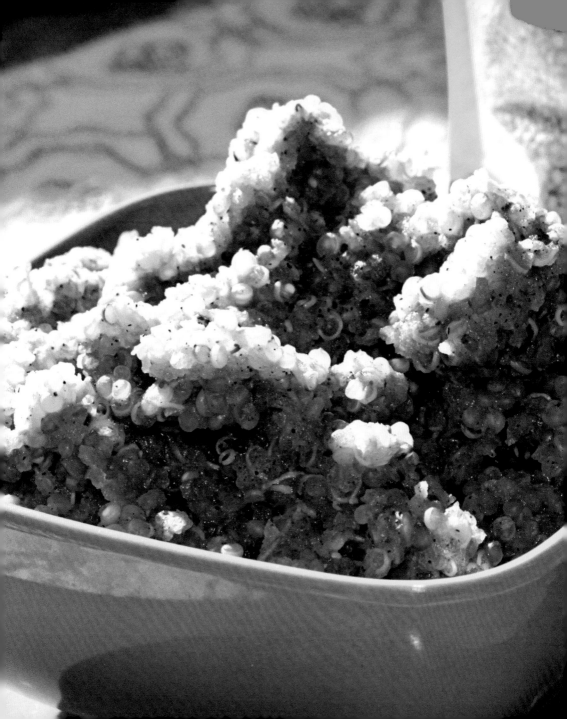

BAKED APPLE BREAD PUDDING OATMEAL

INGREDIENTS:

1 ½ cups vanilla almond milk

1 tsp baking powder

1 tsp cinnamon

dash salt

1 tsp vanilla

1 scoop low-carb vanilla
protein powder

⅓ cup diced Fuji apple

3 Tbsp raisins

2 cups 100% whole-grain bread
ripped into bite-sized pieces

½ cup old-fashioned oats

2 Tbsp slivered almonds

1 cup nonfat vanilla Greek Yogurt,
divided

DIRECTIONS:

Pour almond milk into a bowl. Add baking powder, cinnamon, salt, vanilla, and protein powder. Whisk until thoroughly combined. Add cubed apples, raisins, bread, and oats. Pour into individual oven-proof bowls. Bake at 350 degrees for 30 minutes or until bread pudding is slightly firm to touch and pulls from sides. Remove from oven. Serve each dish with ... cup vanilla Greek Yogurt.

Serving: 4
Prep Time: 3 minutes
Cook Time: 30 minutes

If you know me, you know how much I love bread pudding. During contest prep bread pudding is my cheat of choice.

NUTRITION:

Calories 257 | Fat 4.38g | Sodium 227.52mg | Carbs 37.4g | Fiber 4.17g
Sugars 20.73g | Protein 16.42g

SIMPLE HOMEMADE MUESLI

INGREDIENTS:

¾ cup old-fashioned oats

2 Tbsp toasted wheat germ

4 Tbsp wheat bran

4 Tbsp oat bran

2 Tbsp sunflower seeds

2 Tbsp chopped walnuts

2 Tbsp unsweetened dried
   cranberries

2 Tbsp raisins

DIRECTIONS:

Combine ingredients in a bowl. Store in an airtight container for up to a month.

Serving: 1
Prep Time: 3 minutes
Cook Time: N/A

Here's another healthy muesli option. I love the addition of sunflower seeds.

NUTRITION:

Calories: 261 | Fat: 8.29g | Sodium: 4.75mg | Carbs: 41.78g | Fiber: 6.51g
Sugars: 14.99 | Protein: 8.43g

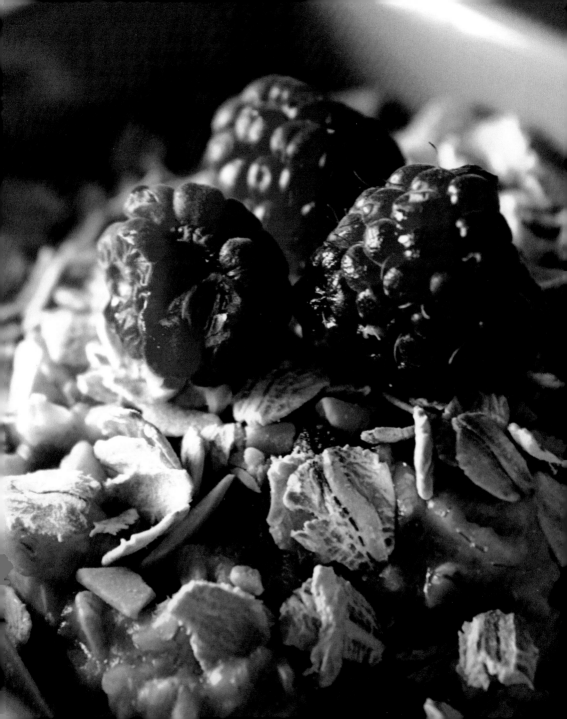

STOVETOP RASPBERRY CRUMBLE OATMEAL

INGREDIENTS:

⅔ cup old-fashioned oats
separated

¼ cup fresh or frozen
raspberries

½ tsp cinnamon

¾ Tbsp chopped almonds

1 cup water

sugar substitute, to taste

Cooking oatmeal on the stovetop is still the old standard. My oatmeal on the stove always comes out thick and creamy whereas with baked oatmeal it tends to rise and cook up.

DIRECTIONS:

Mix 1/2 cup dry oats with 1 cup water and raspberries. Cook on stove on medium heat for 10 minutes or until soft. Move top rack in oven to highest setting. Preheat oven to 400. Toast almonds and remaining oats in oven 3 to 5 minutes or until golden. Pour cooked oatmeal into bowl. Sprinkle with browned oats and almonds. Sweeten with sugar substitute.

Serving: 1
Prep Time: 3 minutes
Cook Time: 10 minutes

NUTRITION:

Calories 250 | Fat 7.07g | Sodium 0mg | Carbs 41.37g | Fiber 8.39g
Sugars 2.77g | Protein 8.07g

BAKED CARAMEL BANANA BREAD PUDDING OATMEAL

INGREDIENTS:

1 ½ cups vanilla almond milk

1 tsp baking powder

1 tsp cinnamon

dash salt

4 Tbsp Torani sugar-free
   Caramel syrup

½ cup nonfat cottage cheese

1 tsp vanilla

1 scoop low-carb vanilla protein powder

2 Tbsp chopped walnuts

1 banana, chopped

2 cups 100% whole-grain bread
   (ripped into bite-sized pieces)

½ cup old-fashioned oats

2 Tbsp brown sugar/Splenda blend, divided

1 cup nonfat vanilla Greek Yogurt, divided

DIRECTIONS:

Pour almond milk into a bowl. Add baking powder, cinnamon, salt, caramel syrup, cottage cheese, vanilla, and protein powder. Whisk until thoroughly combined. Add walnuts, banana, bread, and oats and mix until combined. Pour into 4 individual oven-proof bowls. Sprinkle each bowl with brown sugar/ Splenda blend equally. Bake at 350 degrees for 30 minutes or until bread pudding is slightly firm to touch and pulls from sides. Remove from oven. Serve each dish with ... 1 cup vanilla Greek Yogurt.

Serving: 2   Prep Time: 3 minutes   Cook Time: 30 minutes

NUTRITION:

Calories 263 | Fat 4.5g | Sodium 367.5mg | Carbs 36.63g | Fiber 4.13g
Sugars 19.13g | Protein 19.63g

BAKED PECAN PIE OATMEAL

INGREDIENTS:

½ cup old-fashioned oats

1 cup vanilla almond milk

¼ tsp baking powder

½ tsp vanilla

¼ tsp cinnamon

¼ tsp nutmeg

½ tsp butter extract

¼ tsp maple extract

1 Stevia packet

1 Tbsp chopped pecans

5-10 sprays butter

1 Tbsp brown sugar/Splenda blend

DIRECTIONS:

Combine all but last 3 ingredients in an oven-proof bowl. Bake at 350 degrees for 20 minutes until slightly firm. Meanwhile, chop pecans. Remove oatmeal from oven. Sprinkle oatmeal with chopped pecans and brown sugar/Splenda blend and coat with spray butter. Place back in oven and bake for an additional 10 minutes.

Serving: 1
Prep Time: 3 minutes
Cook Time: 30 minutes

Sometimes I'll add extra pecans if I'm feeling like a cheat. If I'm not, this is about as much as I justify without going too overboard! So good!

NUTRITION:

Calories 368 | Fat 16.79g | Sodium 180.08mg | Carbs 43.51g | Fiber 6.27g
Sugars 13.95g | Protein 6.03g

BANANA CREAM PIE OATMEAL

INGREDIENTS:

2 cups water

dash salt

1 cup old-fashioned oats

½ banana, thinly sliced

¼ cup fat-free sweetened
   condensed milk

1 tsp vanilla

⅔ cup nonfat vanilla Greek Yogurt,
divided

DIRECTIONS:

Bring water and a dash of salt to a boil. Add oats. Let cook for up to 5 minutes or until done. Reduce heat to low. Stir in banana, sweetened condensed milk, and vanilla. Cook for an additional few minutes or until bananas turn to mush. Serve in two bowls, topping each with ⅓ cup nonfat vanilla Greek Yogurt.

Serving: 2
Prep Time: 3 minutes
Cook Time: 30 minutes

Just like Grandma Passey used to make...but oatmeal instead.

NUTRITION:

Calories 34 | Fat 3g | Sodium 80.02mg | Carbs 64.25g | Fiber 5g
Sugars 35.92g | Protein 15.59g

DRIED APPLE QUICK OATS

INGREDIENTS:

½ cup quick oats

½ cup unsweetened 100% apple juice

½ cup water

1 Tbsp golden raisins

1 Tbsp dried apples

dash cinnamon

dash apple pie spice

¼ cup nonfat vanilla Greek Yogurt

DIRECTIONS:

Mix all but last ingredient in a microwavable bowl. Cook on high for 2 to 3 minutes, stirring every 30-45 seconds. When it's thickened to your liking, remove from microwave. Top with yogurt and serve. Sprinkle with additional cinnamon and apple pie spice too if you'd like!

Serving: 1
Prep Time: 3 minutes
Cook Time: 3 minutes

You can also make this recipe with old-fashioned oats on the stove. Just allow yourself a little more time. If you are in a hurry, this is a yummy one to throw together and go!

NUTRITION:

Calories 284 | Fat 3.15g | Sodium 29.41mg | Carbs 57.74g | Fiber 5.04g
Sugars 29.05g | Protein 9.82g

KEY LIME BAKED OATMEAL

INGREDIENTS:

½ cup old-fashioned oats

½ cup vanilla almond milk

½ cup water

½ tsp lime zest

½ tsp vanilla

juice of ½ lime, squeezed dry

¼ tsp baking powder

1 Tbsp brown sugar/Splenda blend

1 square whole-wheat graham cracker

DIRECTIONS:

Combine everything except for brown sugar and graham crackers in an oven-proof bowl. Bake at 350 degrees for 30 minutes or until oatmeal pulls from sides of bowl. Remove from oven. Crumble graham cracker over top and sprinkle with brown sugar/Splenda blend.

Serving: 1
Prep Time: 3 minutes
Cook Time: 30 minutes

Can't get much closer to the real thing!

NUTRITION:

Calories 230 | Fat 5.2g | Sodium 132.5mg | Carbs 38.9g | Fiber 4.7g
Sugars 7.7g | Protein 6g

LEMON APPLE POPPYSEED BAKED OATMEAL

INGREDIENTS:

½ cup old-fashioned oats

¼ tsp baking powder

1 cup water

3 Tbsp unsweetened organic
   applesauce

1 tsp poppy seeds

½ to 1 tsp freshly grated
   lemon zest

sugar substitute, to taste

dash cinnamon

DIRECTIONS:

Combine in an oven-proof
bowl. Bake at 350 degrees for
30 minutes.

Serving: 1
Prep Time: 3 minutes
Cook Time: 30 minutes

My mom used to buy the assorted muffins from Costco when I was younger.
They were a delicious treat. We'd have them as snacks. Little did I know how
unhealthy they were at the time. I created this recipe as a result—reminds
me of the Poppyseed Muffins.

NUTRITION:

Calories 185 | Fat 3g | Sodium 3.75mg | Carbs 32.83g | Fiber: 5.35g
Sugars 4g | Protein 5.05g

MOCK ALMOND JOY OATMEAL

INGREDIENTS:

1 cup vanilla almond milk

½ cup old-fashioned oats

2 Tbsp Torani sugar-free
  Chocolate syrup

½ tsp almond extract

1 Tbsp unsweetened
  shredded coconut

2 Tbsp slivered almonds

dark chocolate chips (optional)

When I was younger Almond Joys were one of my favorite candy bars. Almond Joys and Mounds. Thank goodness almonds are good for you. Add a little coconut and some chocolate sugar-free and calorie-free syrup, and you can almost imagine you're eating the real thing—for breakfast!

DIRECTIONS:

Bring almond milk to a boil. Add oats, reduce heat to medium, and cook for up to 5 minutes until done, stirring occasionally. Reduce heat to low. Stir in 2 Tbsp Torani sugar-free chocolate syrup, almond extract, coconut flakes, and slivered almonds. Cook and stir for 2 minutes more. Pour into a serving dish. Add a few dark chocolate chips if desired.

Serving: 1
Prep Time: 3 minutes
Cook Time: 30 minutes

NUTRITION:

Calories 321 | Fat 17g | Sodium 181.71mg | Carbs 33.17g | Fiber 7.17g
Sugars 2g | Protein 9g

PUMPKIN AND NUT STOVETOP OATMEAL

INGREDIENTS:

½ cup old-fashioned oats

½ cup unsweetened almond milk

½ cup water

⅓ cup pumpkin puree

¼ tsp cinnamon

dash nutmeg

½ Tbsp agave nectar or honey

1 Tbsp chopped walnuts

Another stovetop seasonal favorite.

DIRECTIONS:

Combine in a small saucepan and cook over medium heat for 5 minutes or until most of liquid is absorbed and oatmeal is soft.

Serving: 1

Prep Time: 3 minutes

Cook Time: 10 minutes

NUTRITION:

Calories: 269 | Fat: 8.5g | Sodium 138.33mg | Carbs 43.24g | Fiber 8.83g
Sugars 11.41g | Protein 7.83g

QUICK OATMEAL MIX

INGREDIENTS:

6 cups quick oats

1 ½ cups instant nonfat dried milk

1 cup raisins

½ cup brown sugar/Splenda blend

½ tsp salt

½ Tbsp cinnamon

½ Tbsp nutmeg

½ Tbsp allspice

½ Tbsp ground cloves

This is great to have on hand—already mixed. Just pour out your desired amount, throw it in the microwave, cook, and go!

DIRECTIONS:

For storage: Combine in an airtight container. Shake, cover tightly, and store until needed. To cook: Measure ½ cup of oatmeal mix and place in a microwavable dish. Add 1 cup of water and stir well. Microwave on high, stirring every 30-45 seconds, until cooked to desired consistency. Drizzle with almond milk and serve.

Serving: 12

Prep Time: 3 minutes

NUTRITION:

Calories 251 | Fat 3.18g | Sodium 143.94mg | Carbs 49.88g | Fiber 5.11g
Sugars 22.59g | Protein 6.5g

S'MORES BAKED OATMEAL

INGREDIENTS:

1 cup water

1 envelope hot cocoa mix with mini marshmallows

½ cup old-fashioned oats

dash salt

¼ tsp baking powder

8-10 dark chocolate chips

1 square graham cracker

Walden Farms zero calorie chocolate sauce *(optional)*

Who needs a campfire when you have S'mores baked oatmeal?

DIRECTIONS:

Bring water to a boil in a pot on the stove. Add hot cocoa mix and stir until dissolved. Let cool slightly. Place oats, salt, and baking powder in an oven-proof bowl. Pour hot cocoa on oats. Add dark chocolate chips, distributing evenly throughout oatmeal. Bake at 350 degrees for 30 minutes or until edges pull from sides. Remove oatmeal from oven. Crumble graham cracker over top and serve. Drizzle with Walden Farms chocolate syrup if desired.

Serving: 1
Prep Time: 3 minutes
Cook Time: 30 minutes

NUTRITION:

Calories 283 | Fat 8.2g | Sodium 203.67mg | Carbs 50.4g | Fiber 4.53g
Sugars 18.53g | Protein 5.83g

SPICE CAKE OATMEAL

INGREDIENTS:

½ cup old-fashioned oats

¼ cup unsweetened 100% apple juice

¾ cup water

¼ cup chopped tart green apple

1 Tbsp chopped dates

1 Tbsp raisins

½ Tbsp chopped pecans

¼ tsp ginger

¼ tsp cloves

½ tsp vanilla

agave or honey, to taste *(optional)*

A hearty combination of bakery flavors!

DIRECTIONS:

Combine oats, apple juice, water, fruit, and spices in a pot. Bring to a boil and reduce heat to medium. Continue to cook for 2-3 minutes while stirring until desired consistency. Remove from heat and stir in vanilla. Top oatmeal with chopped pecans and drizzle with agave or honey to your liking.

Serving: 1

Prep Time: 2 minutes

Cook Time: 5 minutes

NUTRITION:

Calories 335 | Fat 8.29g | Sodium 12.11mg | Carbs 61.19g | Fiber 7.85g
Sugars 30.69g | Protein 5.77g

SPIKED RUM AND PEAR QUICK OATS

INGREDIENTS:

½ cup quick oats

1 cup water

½ cup canned pears in light syrup (use both pears and syrup)

1 tsp imitation rum (found in baking aisle)

¼ cup nonfat vanilla Greek Yogurt

½ Tbsp chopped walnuts

I have to admit some of my favorite desserts are a flambé, when they soak the fruit in rum. Why not try it with oatmeal using cooking imitation rum instead? I did, and it's delish!

DIRECTIONS:

Combine oats with 1 cup of water and bring to a boil. Cook until almost done (about 1-2 minutes). Stir in pears (as-is or chopped), light pear juice, and rum extract. Cook over medium heat for one minute more. Pour into a serving dish and top with nonfat vanilla Greek Yogurt and chopped walnuts.

Serving: 1

Prep Time: 3 minutes

Cook Time: 5 minutes

NUTRITION:

Calories 273 | Fat 5g | Sodium 51.35mg | Carbs 44.03g | Fiber 5.75g
Sugars 11.16g | Protein 11.02g

TART BAKED LEMON OATMEAL

INGREDIENTS:

½ cup old-fashioned oats

1 cup water, just shy of

1 Tbsp lemon juice

¼ tsp baking powder

½ tsp lemon peel

1 Tbsp brown sugar/Splenda
   granular

½ tsp vanilla

1 tsp imitation butter extract

agave or honey, to taste *(optional)*

unsweetened almond milk
(optional)

DIRECTIONS:

Combine the above all but last two ingredients in an oven-proof bowl. Bake at 350 degrees for 30 minutes or until oatmeal pulls from sides of bowl. Remove from oven, and serve alone or drizzle with agave or honey and almond milk.

Serving: 1

Prep Time: 3 minutes

Cook Time: 30 minutes

This oatmeal is a nice balance of tart and sweet.

NUTRITION:
Calories 210 | Fat 3g | Sodium 0mg | Carbs 39g | Fiber 4g | Sugars 13g | Protein 5g

STEEL-CUT BREAKFAST BARS WITH FRUIT SAUCE

INGREDIENTS:

Oatmeal Bars:

1 cup unsweetened almond milk

¼ tsp salt

1 tsp vanilla

1 tsp maple extract

½ tsp cinnamon

2 tbsp Flaxseed Ground

1 ½ cups steel cut oats

3 cups water

¼ cup Splenda/Brown Sugar blend

Fruit Sauce:

2 tbsp agave syrup

3 oz unsweetened cranberries

3 oz golden raisins

¼ cup Splenda/Brown Sugar Blend

½ tsp cinnamon

1 ¾ cups water

¾ cup sugar-free maple syrup

DIRECTIONS:

Fruit: combine water, fruit, sugar, and spices in a pot; bring to a boil. Reduce heat, and simmer until thick.

Bars: combine water, milk, brown sugar, ½ teaspoon cinnamon, vanilla, maple extract, and salt in a pot. Boil over medium-high heat; stir in oats and flaxseed. Reduce heat, and simmer for 20 minutes. Spoon into an 11x7 baking dish coated with spray. Cover and chill until set. Serve with fruit and maple syrup.

Serving: 8   Prep Time: 3 minutes   Cook Time: 30 minutes

NUTRITION:

Calories 217 | Fat 3g | Sodium 113.67mg | Carbs 43.19g | Fiber 4.94g
Sugars 16.53g | Protein 4.36g

A Q&A WITH JENNY GROTHE

....

What supplements do you take?

I'm religious about taking my multi-vitamins; I take a good multi, B-complex, and Vitamins C, D, and E. To help with muscle recovery and building, I also take creatine, glutamine powder, and BCAAs. All are natural. A lot of women are afraid to take creatine––like it's a dirty word. Taking the right dosage is completely safe and helps to maximize your efforts in the gym.

How do you maintain your muscle tone while prepping for a marathon?

I get asked this question all the time. Everyone has a different opinion on it. For me? I simply ask myself, am I willing to give up lifting weights while I train for a marathon? The answer is no. Am I willing to give up running while I'm training for a show? Again, the answer is no. Both are extremely important to me. I might cut back my running a little (drop the long runs and stick to three to four miles each time instead), but I won't give up running altogether. It's just not me, and it's not worth it to me. Others will undoubtedly feel differently about it. If training for a competition is your number-one priority, then you might want to stick to other forms of cardio, or shorter bursts of running (think sprints). If you are looking to enjoy your hobbies (all of them), I just say do what feels enjoyable. To me that's really what it's all about anyway.

Do I need to take steroids in order to compete in Figure?

This is such a touchy subject. I've often wondered the same thing, especially when I was first starting out—and keep in mind I'm still fairly "green." I've only been an active part of this industry for three years. I wanted the beefy arms and the rounded shoulders. I wanted everything to pop, and I wanted it all now. I wondered how everyone else got those arms. I worked so hard and it seemed like it made little difference, of course, in reality I'd only been at it for a short period of time. Essentially, I found myself wondering if I needed to take something in order to compete.

I never have.

Competitors on the message boards would tell me, "Be patient. Give it time." That's what I have done. Slowly but surely with hard work, determination, creatine, glutamine, protein, and BCAAs, my muscle tone has improved. I now see peaks where I saw valleys. It's taken three years to go from where I was to where I am now. It doesn't happen overnight. That's just not realistic. And I still have a long way to go. I know what I want to look like, and I'm definitely not there. But I have improved.

I still compete without.

In saying that, I would also venture to say that some competitors do cross that line.

Work hard. Train hard. Eat right. Supplement safely. Know what you may or may not be up against. If you live in a state that's extremely competitive where you think you might be up against unfair circumstances, opt for natural shows. The NPC offers all-natural shows, and the NGA is all natural.

Above all, do it for you and don't worry about what others are doing. Focus on your body and bring your personal best to each show you do and enjoy the experience.

How do you get so lean?

I'd like to say it's as easy as simple clean eating and exercise. That is a huge part of it, but that's not the whole story. It comes down to genetics, your body, your metabolism, your age—all of that. I do tend to stay relatively lean throughout the year, but I carry it in my abs. I'll sometimes look at someone else and think, "How does she get her abs so tight?" But she might carry it in her arms or in her thighs. It's all part of our genetic makeup. Just the same, to be the lean you you're meant to be, eat clean. Eat simply. Eat whole grains, fruits, vegetables, and lean proteins. The cleaner you eat, the leaner you'll be. There's no secret. Just know that you might lean out differently than someone else, and that's okay.

How does your diet differ when training for a marathon than when you're training for a competition?

This question ties in to the one I answered before. I never give up one for the other. That would not make me happy. I would sorely miss one without the other. I always lift and run. When I was training for my most recent marathon,

I alternated. I had a runner's program I was following for my marathon. As my runs during the week increased, I started alternating gym and running days. For example, I'd run Tuesdays, Thursdays, and Saturdays. I'd hit the gym Mondays, Wednesdays, and Fridays. Saturdays would be my long run, and then Sunday I'd rest. The days I'd hit the gym I'd still cross-train. I'd do something that was challenging, got my heart rate up, and worked up a good sweat. When I'm not training for a marathon I like to do both when possible. My ideal day is to run three to four miles first thing in the morning and then hit the gym after my kiddo is in school. That's not always possible though, so I fit in what I can when I can. Somehow I always seem to be prepared come comp or marathon time.

How much protein should I be consuming to build muscle?

Again, ask two different people, and you'll get two different answers. I've heard and read everything from .7 grams of protein to every pound of bodyweight to 2 grams of protein to every pound of bodyweight. Me personally? I shoot for about 1.5 grams of protein for every pound of bodyweight. You need to also consider how hard you are training. If you consume too much protein and are not training enough to support the need for the extra protein, your body will store the excess protein as fat. So, if you feel you train moderately, maybe stick toward the lower end (.8 grams per pound of bodyweight). If you are training hard, and lifting heavy and building muscle is your goal, set your number higher. Here's an example: for most of the year I try to stay around 120 pounds. If I plan on 1.5 grams of protein per pound of bodyweight, I should be consuming no fewer than 180 grams of protein a day.

What's your typical meal plan?

I am a simple eater. I try to plan ahead, and I often times have the same thing for breakfast, snacks, and lunches day after day. I'll change up my dinner most nights. This might not sound appealing to you, and it doesn't always sound good to me either. When I started training for comps my view of food changed. I'd still have cravings, but I wanted food more for fuel than for taste. I'm still the same way...for the most part. I like to eat things I enjoy, but it really doesn't bother me to have the same foods all the time. Crazy, I know. I'll usually have a low-carb, low-fat protein shake immediately following my workout. For breakfast I will cook a baked oatmeal with cottage cheese and supplement it with hardboiled egg whites. I'll have tuna and a piece of Ezekiel bread for my snack, and then chicken or fish with steamed spinach for lunch. Afternoon snack consists of an apple and some PB2 along with some egg whites. I usually have a yummy salad for dinner. At night before bed I always make a frozen protein shake. That's it. Simple. Routine. Works for me. The key is figuring out what works for you. It also might depend on what your mood is. Some days you might feel like cooking all day. I go through that. Others you just want to pull stuff out in a hurry and get it down. In my opinion the key is to plan, prepare, and decide ahead of time what options you have. That way you won't find yourself rummaging through the pantry hoping for a healthy treat.

How often should I be eating?

You should be eating every two to three hours. It's that simple. If you miss a meal (which I hope you don't), don't try to make up for it with your next meal. Excess carbs, calories, and proteins are stored as fat. Your body only needs so much at any given meal. Go over that number, and it's wasted. That's the idea behind eating every two to three hours. It's not so much to make you happier but rather to provide the right types of fuel to your body when your body needs it. You're constantly giving your body the fuel it needs to go...and grow.

What's in your fridge?

When I first starting losing weight, so many of my friends and neighbors wanted to know what was in my fridge. It was almost embarrassing, but I guess we can learn a lot by studying what we store in our fridges and our pantries. So, here's what's in mine. I always stock up on fresh fruits and vegetables. I love apples, oranges, bananas, grapefruit, strawberries, and blueberries. I stock up on what's in season. I really love salads, so I keep all the fixings. You'll always find romaine, leafy greens, spinach, tomatoes, avocados, carrots, onions, butternut squash, zucchini, asparagus, and green beans in my fridge. I always stock up on VOSKOS nonfat Greek Yogurt, nonfat cottage cheese, fresh eggs, chicken, flank steak, and tuna. I prep as much as I can in advance. After prepping, I store my cooked foods in large Tupperware to keep until I eat them. This is especially true for chicken, fish, flank, squash, and yams. I can usually make prepped foods last three to four days--which is great. That means no needless time-consuming cooking for those days. As for beverages? Water and Propel packets.

What's your favorite protein powder?

This changes. Right now my very favorite all-purpose protein powder is Topform's Vanilla protein powder. It's low-calorie, nonfat, and low-carb. To round out my top three, I'd say Isopure's Zero-Carb Cookies and Cream and BSN's Fresh Cinnamon Roll Lean Dessert. If I have those three protein powders on hand, I really don't need any others. The reality though? I'm a protein powder junkie, and I love to try new flavors. The ones I don't like? I give to my husband. Shh!

What's your favorite post-workout meal?

As a general rule of thumb, I try to have a protein shake (powder and water) in a mixer ready to go immediately following my workout. Some say your window of opportunity to take in your protein is 30 minutes––others say an hour. I say play it safe and have it ready as you walk out the door of the gym. Post-workout is a great time to have some quick simple sugars too. This helps draw the protein in. So, I'll have some berries, a half of banana, or a handful of chopped dates. I make sure my post-workout meal has somewhere between 20-30 grams of protein. I'll then go home and prepare my Baked Oatmeal.

How did you find your motivation?

I found my motivation in a pair of men's swim trunks. It really was the icing on the cake. Bad experiences were mounting, and I'd had enough. I found my motivation in my desire to not have to wear men's trunks, or XL tops, or not be able to hike, or have to avoid the camera. I was tired of hiding in oversized, baggy clothes. That's where my initial motivation came from. I channeled those experiences into drive.

Why was this time different from the other times when you lost your weight?

Something clicked. I don't know how else to say it. They say it takes three weeks to make a new habit. I think that applied at the beginning, but the real commitment had to come from within. I'd worked out before. I'd been a member at other gyms. I'd trained. I have actually seen progress at other times in my life. But I always gave up, gave in, or somehow let all my progress fade away. This time it was mental. I really did tell myself (and continue to tell myself) that giving up wasn't an option. I never wanted to be that unhealthy again. As I dropped my weight, I got rid of every reminder of how big I was. I no longer wanted to hang on to my fat jeans just in case. Just in case of what? I'd need them? I didn't want that. So, I trained hard, started eating healthier, became more active socially, and revamped my closet and drawers. I wasn't going to give in to excuse or old habits. That's what was different. It didn't stop when I lost my weight though. It's a daily struggle. Every day I am forced to make decisions––decisions that can either keep me on the right path or set me back. It's the small daily choices that keep you strong or just the opposite.

What's your workout schedule like and how long do you train?

I'm a gym junkie, but I'm not near as bad as I used to be. I used to train anywhere from two to three hours by the time I'd get my weight-training and cardio in. I thought more was better. There really is such a thing as over-training. Now I weight train for 30-45 minutes and do cardio for 30-45 minutes. I'm never in the gym longer than 90 minutes anymore. When I have my iPod and my gym gloves on, I mean business. I rarely stop and talk with anyone. That's part of the beauty of training so early in the morning. Most people at the gym at 5 a.m. mean business too. They aren't there to socialize. Go any later in the morning and not only is it busier, but there are a lot more distractions–– whether you want them or not. Right now my winter workout split is: Monday:

Shoulders and Cardio; Tuesday: Back and Cardio; Wednesday: Glutes, Abs, and Cardio; Thursday: Bis and Tris and Cardio; Friday: either Shoulders or Back (2nd session for the week) and Cardio; and Saturday: Legs and Cardio. I'll fit in an extra ab workout here and there. I don't train my chest much anymore. It contributed to some muscle imbalances, so I am trying to pull my shoulders back and strengthen my back. Cardio consists mostly of running, the stepmill, and treadmill walking at a steep incline. Once spring hits, I'll change my schedule again so I can include more outside running.

How long did it take you before you saw results?

I saw results within three months. I remember because I'd started back to the gym in September 2007, and we headed to Hawaii for Christmas just three short months later. I'd dropped from a size 12-14 to a size 10, and I felt on top of the world. That translated to 20 lbs, and I felt hot for the first time in I don't know how long. Keep in mind, I read the entire Twilight series on the stationary bike at the gym. That didn't hurt. As long as I kept my mind active, the time flew, and the fat melted away.

Did you always enjoy cooking?

Yes. In a strange way it connects me to my mom. I was always so proud of her growing up. I loved having my friends over because she was such an amazing cook, and I knew her meals were different than meals in most of my friends' homes. She wasn't about the quick fix. She was about a full-meal experience. She would also set the table right down to tablecloths, placemats, and real napkins. It was a dining experience, not just dinner. I think of her when I'm in the kitchen. So much of what I learned I learned from my mom. I love to try new things all the time—that is one thing that's different from my mom. Mom always enjoyed preparing tried-and-true recipes for friends and family. Me? I'll try something completely new on a whim and hope for the best when friends and family come over. Most of the time it turns out; other times... uh, we look forward to dessert. Mom says I get the "experimental gene" from my grandma. Ha ha!

Does oatmeal cause gas?

Yes it can. One of the strongest benefits of eating oatmeal is that it contains fiber, which helps to keep your system moving. With more fiber in the diet comes the possibility of more gas as well. The more you eat, the more likely the problem. That's why it's so important to keep your fluid intake up, so you can help move it through your system.

Do you ever get sick of oatmeal?

No. It's been three years of having it nearly every day, and I haven't yet. If anything, I like it more now than I did then. Must be the Baked Oatmeal.

RECOMMENDED READING AND SITES

For Training:

Oxygen Magazine – http://www.oxygenmag.com

Muscle & Fitness Hers Magazine - http://www.muscleandfitnesshers.com/

Making the Cut, Jillian Michaels

Strength Training Anatomy, Frederic Delavier

101 Workouts for Women, Muscle & Fitness HERS

Bodybuilding.com, www.bodybuilding.com

Runners World Magazine - http://www.runnersworld.com/

4 Months to a 4 Hour Marathon, Dave Kuehls

For Diet and Recipes:

Recipes for Gals in Figure and Bodybuilding, Facebook

Jen-Fit's Fitness and Recipe Blog - jen-fit-training.blogspot.com/

Clean Eating Magazine - cleaneatingmag.com/minisite/ce_index.htm

Cooking Light Magazine - cookinglight.com/magazine/

The Eat Clean Diet, Tosca Reno

The Eat Clean Diet Cookbook, Tosca Reno

Eat This Not That – The No-Diet Weight Loss Solution!, David Zinczenko

Eat This Not That – Supermarket Survival Guide, David Zinczenko

Eat This Not That – Restaurant Survival Guide, David Zinczenko

Eat Right Guide, Men's Health

Master Your Metabolism, Jillian Michaels

Hungry Girl 200 under 200, Lisa Lillien

Fresh Food Fast, Cooking Light, Oxmoor House

For Competing:

Oxygen Magazine – oxygenmag.com

Muscle & Fitness Hers Magazine - muscleandfitnesshers.com

Sioux Country – siouxcountry.com

Hardbody – hardbody.com

Bodybuilding.com – bodybuilding.com

ABOUT THE AUTHOR

Jenny's life changed during the fall of 2007. That's when she decided to shed 60 pounds, trade unhealthy habits for good ones, and start leading her life rather than letting her life lead her.

It was at that time she learned about clean eating. Since then she has sought out and tried hundreds of recipes. Finding that most of her tried-and-true recipes of the past needed tweaking in order to be healthy, she discovered a new passion: experimenting. She is now the author and administrator of the popular Facebook Fan Page, "Recipes for Gals in Figure and Bodybuilding," which boasts more than 17,000 fans and grows by an average of 500 each week.

It was through the countless suggestions from her fans, who loved her daily recipes, that she finally decided to create a cookbook.

Always on the lookout for a good recipe, you can find Jenny in the kitchen, browsing magazines, scouring the Web, and leafing through cookbooks. That's where she finds her inspiration.

When she's not trying a new recipe or creating her own, you can find Jenny either at the gym or laying down some miles on road. As an amateur figure competitor, Jenny loves the hard work, determination, and dedication it takes to compete on stage. In the three short years she's been competing, she's brought home 5 trophies.

Jenny's new favorite quote reads, "My body is my trophy. My placing does not define me."

She also loves long-distance running and recently qualified for the Boston Marathon, which she'll be running in 2011.

As a sponsored athlete for Topform, Jenny continues to train and study in the area of health and fitness as she strives to help those around her.

Jenny is thankful for the journey she's been on and looks forward to what the future holds, believing that all things are possible.

Prior to being a homemaker, Jenny spent 15 years in Sales and Marketing, where she had the privilege to learn from the best, live abroad, and travel throughout Europe.

Now, as a stay-at-home mom, Jenny is most thankful for her family. She married her sweetheart 19 years ago and since then they've adopted two beautiful boys, Dakota (9) and Zane (16 months).

As an active member in the Church of Jesus Christ of Latter-day Saints, Jenny believes in serving and helping others. She hopes this cookbook will provide not only new competitors, but oatmeal lovers everywhere with new and tasty ways to prepare one of her favorite foods...oats.

May the oatmeal inspiration never cease to end.

RECIPE INDEX

Symbols
6-Grain Blueberry Baked Oatmeal 115

A
Apple Peanut Butter Baked Oatmeal 136
Apple Pie Quinoa 151

B
Baked Apple Bread Pudding Oatmeal 158
Baked Apple Pie Oatmeal 75
Baked Banana Oatmeal in Rum 76
Baked Caramel Banana Bread Pudding
Oatmeal 162
Baked Pecan Pie Oatmeal 163
Banana Bread Baked Oatmeal 81
Banana Bread Crockpot Steel Cut Oats 82
Banana Cream Pie Oatmeal 164
Black Forest Baked Oatmeal 84
Blueberry Cheesecake Baked Oatmeal 122
Blueberry Latte Baked Oatmeal 124
Brown Sugar and Baked Date Oatmeal 83
Brown Sugar Pineapple Baked Oatmeal 87

C
Caramel Apple Pie Oatmeal 89
Cheesy Peach-on-Peach Baked Oatmeal 127
Cherry Cranberry Tart Baked Oatmeal 125
Chocolate-Drizzled PB Toffee Baked Oatmeal
88
Choconana Baked Oatmeal 137
Cinnamon Chocolate Chip Baked Oatmeal
128
Cinnamon Coconut Granola 147
Creamy Chocolate Pumpkin Baked Oatmeal
131
Creamy Pumpkin Cranberry Baked Oatmeal
129
Creamy Rice Hot Protein Cereal 152
Crockpot Company Fruit Oatmeal 139

D
Dark Cherry Baked Oatmeal 91
Dirty Chai Baked Oatmeal 90
Dried Apple Quick Oats 165
Dried Cranberry Baked Oatmeal 92
Dried Pineapple and Cherry Baked Oatmeal 140
Dry Cinnamon Oatmeal Snack 153

F
Fruity Almond Muesli 154

G
Ginger Pumpkin Baked Oatmeal 133
Golden Fig Baked Oatmeal 94

H
Hearty Homemade Baked Oatmeal 97

J
Juicy Berry Baked Oatmeal 100

K
Key Lime Baked Oatmeal 166

L
Lemon Apple Poppyseed Baked Oatmeal 167

M
Maple Pumpkin Baked Oatmeal 134
Mock Almond Joy Oatmeal 168
My Favorite Crockpot Oatmeal 142

N
Nutty Oatmeal Breakfast Bars 108

O
Oatmeal Protein Shake 155
Orange Coconut Baked Oatmeal 99
Orange Oat Pancakes 103
Overnight Mixed-Grain Oatmeal 141
Overnight No-Cook Citrus Steel Cut Oats 105
Overnight No-Cook Peach Oatmeal 107

P
Peach Cobbler Baked Oatmeal 101
Peach Strudel Baked Oatmeal 144
Peanut Butter Baked Oatmeal W/ Carob Chips 110

Peanut Butter Banana Split Baked Oatmeal 112
Pumpkin and Nut Stovetop Oatmeal 169
Pumpkin Pie Baked Oatmeal 135

Q
Quick Oatmeal Mix 170
Quinoa for Breakfast 156

R
Raspberry and Cream Cheese Baked Oatmeal 145
Raspberry Cheesecake Baked Oatmeal 111

S
Simple Homemade Muesli 159
S'mores Baked Oatmeal 171
Soaked Oats 117
Spice Cake Oatmeal 172
Spiked Rum and Pear Quick Oats 173
Steel-Cut Breakfast Bars with Fruit Sauce 175
Stovetop Raspberry Crumble Oatmeal 161
Strawberries and Cream Baked Oatmeal 119

T
Tart Baked Lemon Oatmeal 174
Tart Cherry and Blueberry Baked Oatmeal 146
Tart Strawberry Rhubarb Baked Oatmeal 79
The 1st Baked Blueberry Oatmeal 121
Tropical Baked Oatmeal 148